Preventing Menopause

Stopping Ovarian Failure Before It Starts

Preventing Menopause

Stopping Ovarian Failure Before It Starts

Beth Rosenshein

Foreword by Dr. Elena A. Christofides, VP of the American
Association of Clinical Endocrinologists (Ohio Valley Chapter)

Preventing Menopause

Cover and Text Design: Anita Janik-Jones
Cover Image: istockphoto.com

Important Notice:
The purpose of this book is to educate. It is sold with the understanding that the author and publisher shall have neither liability nor responsibility for any injury caused or alleged to be caused directly or indirectly by the information contained in this book. While every effort has been made to ensure its accuracy, the book's contents should not be construed as medical advice. Each person's health needs are unique. To obtain recommendations appropriate to your particular situation, please consult a qualified healthcare provider.

978-0-9889460-0-2

ABOUT THE AUTHOR

Beth Rosenshein is an electrical/bio-medical engineer and is very familiar with medical research. She holds two United States patents, one for a unique design of a vaginal speculum, and one for a clever urinary collection device specifically designed for women. Beth discovered and documented an important drug interaction between esomeprazole (Nexium®) and testosterone. Her findings were published in a case study in The American Journal of the Medical Sciences in May 2004. She petitioned the FDA in August 2003 to change the labeling on hormone products. The petition was granted in September 2004. Beth is also a wife and mother and lives in Boulder, Colorado.

This book is dedicated to my Grandma Fanny,
a suffragette who taught me that every woman's vote counts

ACKNOWLEDGEMENTS

I would like to thank those closest to me, those who believed in me and supported my goal of one day making menopause optional. I especially want to thank my mother, Barbara Diamond Wilson, for always encouraging me and enduring my life-long inquisitiveness.

I would like to thank those who read my book as I was writing it and gave me invaluable feedback (listed in alphabetical order): Elizabeth Anton, M.D.; Nechama Batt-Michelson; Lisa Behar; Bob Bonds, R.Ph.; Rebecca Clark; Robin Cohn; Jane Courage; Scott Eberly, M.D.; Lorre Goldberg; Ron Kornfeld; Stephanie Mailman; Susan Matalon; Anthony McLaughlin, D.D.S.; Rita Rosenshein; Leon Speroff, M.D.; Danya Sterner; Cricket Stimson; Liz Thayer; Laura Wall; and Libby Yuskaitis. Of course, thanks to my Mah-Jongg friends, Erin, Lesley, Sarah and Shelley, who on a weekly basis make me laugh and remind me what is important and what isn't.

I'd like to thank Christine Kernick-Fletcher, the librarian at our local public library. This book would not have been possible without her tremendous efforts. She obtained hundreds of articles that would have been difficult for me to obtain myself. I would also like to thank Caroline Pincus, my book doctor. Caroline helped guide me through the world of publishing and I appreciate all her encouragement and advice.

I would like to thank Elena Christofides, M.D. for her medical review of my book. I deeply appreciate all of her insights and suggestions. I would like to thank my publisher and my team at Your Health Press, for their invaluable help and feedback.

To Leon, my husband, friend and lover—a truly beautiful person—who worked alongside me and helped make this book a reality. I am forever grateful for your love, devotion and inspiration.

Let ours be the last generation to suffer menopause.

TABLE OF CONTENTS

How the Levels of Ovarian Hormones Change Over Time
Risk of Birth Defects
Birth Control
Protecting Your Ovaries

How to Restore Normal Ovarian Hormonal Balance
Define Your Goals
Ovarian Hormone Products
Normalizing Ovarian Function

What I Found
The Goals of the WHI
What the WHI Actually Did

Ovarian Specialists
Understanding Your Laboratory Report

My Journey Continues
The Future of Menopause... For Ourselves, Our Daughters and Our Granddaughters

Finding a Doctor Who Can Help You
How to Find a Doctor or Other Healthcare Professional
Finding a Compounding Pharmacy
Recommended Reading

FOREWORD

Elena A. Christofides, M.D.

Dr. Elena Christofides is a board certified endocrinologist who is listed on the website of "Top Docs" in Columbus, Ohio, where she is now in private practice. She did her training at Ohio State University (Columbus), residency at Mount Carmel Medical Center and fellowship at Louisiana State University (New Orleans). She sits on several medical advisory boards, is a clinical instructor, and is Vice President of the American Association of Clinical Endocrinologists (Ohio Valley Chapter). For more information, visit Dr. Christofides' website: www.endocrinology-associates.com.

Menopausal women today face a daunting array of available information. This information has been designed to help them make the transition to the next phase of their lives and yet, unfortunately, much of it is contradictory. As an endocrinologist, it has never made sense to me that we do not give back what the body—such a complex organism—has lost. The endocrine system is intricately balanced, and the loss of one hormone, let alone several, can have serious consequences for any patient. Some women feel this very acutely in their peri-menopause, the time when their ovaries are slowing down. Clearly, educating patients takes precedence in every discussion regarding what has alternately been regarded as a saving grace and the next great evil—hormone therapy. In fact, I have found that it has become more difficult in my practice to counsel women regarding their hormone needs in this climate, which has been heavily influenced by too little information, and too much media hype.

When I was asked to review Preventing Menopause, I wasn't sure that we needed yet another book in the mix. Once I started reading however, I realized that this particular book could provide a "missing link." In it I found much of the information that I was already presenting to my patients in an effort to give them a balanced portrayal of all the risks and benefits that lie before them in their quest to remain healthy in the menopausal period. I also found that Beth Rosenshein captured the nuances of the science; ultimately she presents it in a way that will enable the menopausal woman to navigate the maze of options available to her.

I hope women and their loved ones use the information in this book to help them make a reasoned, informed plan that will address what is happening to them in this often difficult time. And for the women who seem to make this transition relatively unscathed, it is my hope that they learn just how important it is to remain abreast of the changes that are happening in their bodies, regardless of whether or not they feel them.

INTRODUCTION

Until confronted with menopause I never really gave it much thought. I accepted that I would one day go thorough "the change" just like every other woman. The only thing I knew of menopause was that a woman had hot flashes for a short time and then her life went back to normal, except that she would no longer be able to have a baby. I really thought life would be the same after menopause as it was before. I was in for a rude awakening.

At age 43 I began experiencing changes I was completely unprepared for. My sexual response was completely gone, and after several months I realized that it wasn't coming back. I needed to find out how this happened, if this was normal, and how to adapt to this change. I was baffled. At the time I had no idea that how I was feeling was caused by menopause, which I later learned was complete ovarian failure. I also discovered that it might be possible to prevent or delay this failure. I had no idea that menopause might be optional.

But as I pored over thousands of medical studies and discovered that it might be possible to make menopause optional, I knew I had to write a book. Originally, I planned on writing solely about the use of bio-identical hormones taken to recreate pre-menopausal hormone levels—as opposed to the non-identical hormones such as Premarin™ and Provera™ used in the most commonly prescribed form of Hormone Replacement Therapy (HRT) in an attempt to restore pre-menopausal sexual response. But as I learned more and more about ovarian function, I discovered that as we age we lose our eggs at a faster and faster rate, thus hastening the onset of ovarian failure, and that it may be possible to significantly delay this failure by better managing the eggs with which we are born. Contrary to what nearly every woman—and her doctor—believes, I became convinced that ovarian failure is not inevitable.

I then had to ask: While it may be possible to prevent menopause, is it wise? Are their risks involved? Would there be sufficient health benefits to extend the function of the ovaries until old age? Would birth control be necessary for older women? Is pregnancy a risk for a woman in her 50's, 60's, or 70's? I had to prove to myself that extending the life of the ovaries would not harm a woman's health. *I did.* Through research, I confirmed that restoring a woman's ovarian function through the use of small doses of key hormones (in bio-identical form) can dramatically lower her risk of breast cancer as well as heart disease. I saw that it was possible that the risk of birth defects in babies of older women would likely decrease as well. I found that ovaries contribute a great deal to a woman's overall sense of well-being, and contribute to the functioning of every other organ in her body. Unlike the loss of an appendix, the ovaries' absence is *felt*. Ovaries are not just reproductive organs. They are vital organs, which influence the well-being of every other organ in a woman's body, and thus are important to her overall health. You deserve to know this.

I hope this book will help you see that menopause can be prevented only if you and your doctor (see chapter 2) work towards this goal together. Your doctor will need to know how to help you regulate ovarian function, as well as which medications could derail your efforts.

Very low doses of hormones are needed to regulate ovarian function. I know that hormones have gotten a bad reputation in the last few years, especially due to the findings of the Women's Health Initiative (WHI). As I explain in chapter 6, the hormone replacement therapy used in the WHI study *did not recreate the hormones made by the ovaries, nor is standard HRT based on ovarian function*. These misperceptions are widely shared. The hormones given to the women in the study, standard HRT for over half a century, created a hormonal environment that a woman would not normally experience in her lifetime, either before or after ovarian failure. Understanding the goal of the Women's Health Initiative, as well as how and why particular hormones were chosen, will help you understand the failure of this clinical trial.

Many people are intimidated by the idea of "tinkering" with their hormones. The fact is, this is not really "tinkering" but replacing what the ovaries once produced themselves. The small doses involved are perfectly safe, and are really no different from the treatments doctors use every day to treat any other declining organ in the body in order to help it work at its optimal level. As I will show, there is nothing here to fear.

I am an electrical/bio-medical engineer and am very familiar with medical research. I hold two United States patents, one for a unique design of vaginal speculum, and one for a clever urinary collection device specifically designed for women. I discovered and documented an important drug interaction between esomeprazole (Nexium™) and testosterone. My findings were published in a case study in *The American Journal of the Medical Sciences* in May 2004. I petitioned the FDA in August 2003 to change the labeling on hormone products. The petition was granted in September 2004.

I am also a wife and mother. I wrote this book as much for my children as for myself. I want them to have a better future. Together we can make the future better for our children and ourselves.

The more we know about our bodies, the better equipped we are to help them stay healthy.

CHAPTER ONE

CHANGING THE WAY WE THINK

The right frame of mind is important when embarking on a journey like menopause. For me, the most important thing was to understand what was happening to my body, and what if anything could be done about it. Like everyone else, at the beginning I assumed that menopause was inevitable, and that I would adjust to it. By the time I arrived at my destination, I had learned that ovarian failure takes a tremendous toll on the entire body. I had also come to the understanding that women's bodies work best with ovarian function. I realized that something needed to be done about preventing ovarian failure.

In April 2003 I began a journey that I never envisioned I would take, and life as I knew it would never be the same. My relationship with my husband was dramatically affected, as was my relationship with my four children. Gone was the spontaneous affection I shared with my husband, and the joy I felt just looking at my children. I was 43 years old and I was lost. I questioned how my husband could have such blind devotion to me when I no longer had patience with him. I questioned how I could parent so many children when I felt overwhelmed almost constantly, and when I no longer experienced the joy of just being in the same room with them. I felt isolated from my life. I missed my husband and my children even though they were right in front of me. I thought I was losing my mind.

I remember one night in particular as I sat on the edge of my bed and realized that for two months I had been unable to make love to my husband. I had noticed that my sexual response had been declining for about six months, but for the last two months I had been unable to respond to any sexual stimuli. I made an appointment with my gynecologist to find out what had happened. After a few blood tests she told me that my ovaries were resting, and that they might not wake up. "Resting" ovaries means that there are periods of little or no ovarian function where hormones levels are very low, interspersed with periods of normal function.[1] She told me that menopause could occur anytime within the next 10 years. Then she offered me an estradiol patch. She also offered me testosterone to improve my sexual response. I had no idea what estradiol was. I asked her why she hadn't given me Premarin™, the estrogen pill (used in the Women's Health Initiative). She gave me a puzzled look and said: "Why take away when you only have to put it back?" I was in a rush, as she was, and was unable to ask for an explanation of this cryptic response.

I went home, put on my patch, and began to research the menopausal transition. Within minutes I was feeling "in the mood" again and called my husband home from work to celebrate the good news. This little patch was working! For two days we both basked in the bliss of making love again. Then, inexplicably, my response went away. How could this have happened? How cruel! How could a patch work for two days and then stop? I was devastated. I wanted my life back so badly.

So I went out and bought several books on menopause and read them as quickly as I could. The books reinforced the fact that what I was experiencing was a natural and normal process, and that my body would adjust. I'd feel like myself again. I looked forward to that happening. I had not had a menstrual flow in nearly three months. I was different—not in a good way—and it was affecting my whole family. I was looking for answers and not finding them. I thought if only I could have a normal menstrual cycle, I'd feel good again. I didn't miss blood flow per se, but I knew that after I had my period I always felt better. I just wanted to feel better. I just wanted my life back. I just wanted to be able to feel my husband's touch and enjoy the smell of his skin again. I wanted the pillow talk that now eluded me. I was devastated to realize that we were no longer lovers; rather, we'd become little more than roommates. I cried when I realized that were we to stay together, we'd live a life without the blessing of intimacy. I could find no peace. I could find no solace. I needed answers. My life was literally falling apart. How could this be "normal" or "natural?" I was not transitioning well.

I went back to the bookstore and bought several more books by known and respected authors. I was spending a small fortune on books! Still, I couldn't find the answers I was looking for. I was supposed to be fine. According to these authors, well-respected medical doctors, I would adjust in time, and sexual functioning would once again return. Meanwhile I was dutifully wearing my estradiol patch—and lovemaking still wasn't possible. What was happening? I went to my internist, a very compassionate and knowledgeable doctor, but he had no answers. Maybe I was under stress; maybe it was the kids or my husband's demanding work schedule; maybe it would just take time. In order to remain close to my husband, I needed, at least periodically, the connection of sex. I was so lonely. I felt like I was only going through the motions of life.

Months passed and I was miserable. My entire family was miserable. My husband was worried about me and truly did all he could to be supportive. Yet, right before my very eyes, powerless to stop it, my life was slipping away. The little patch was doing nothing for me as far as I could tell. I bought several more books on menopause and began to see a pattern. These doctors were nothing more than cheerleaders. The books repeated the same bromides over and over again: wisdom was coming my way, intimacy would return, and life would again be normal. So what was different about me? Why wasn't anything changing for the better? My breasts hurt with spark-like sensations, my skin was dry, and my mind was foggy. My whole life had become overwhelming.

Around this time, reports of problems with the Women's Health Initiative were on the news nearly every week. These reports claimed that hormone replacement therapy (HRT) actually *increased* breast cancer and heart disease rates, albeit just slightly. They also claimed that quality of life was *not* enhanced by taking standard HRT, and neither was sexual functioning. I became despondent over the thought that taking hormones would not improve my life—and that they might even make it worse. Every time a news report came out about another negative effect of standard HRT I literally felt sick. Not only was I stuck in a life with no relief in sight, I was getting confirmation from important clinical studies about how miserable the future would be for me, my husband and my children. I'd look at other women in their 40's, 50's, 60's and 70's—women who appeared to be unaffected by menopause—and I'd wonder why I was such a crybaby.

Needless to say, the books on menopause were of no use to me. I barely understood how the ovaries worked, and why some women entered "the change" sooner or handled it better than others. I remember watching a show on the Discovery channel called "The Libido." The show reinforced the notion that sex is possible after ovarian failure, and is not related to ovarian function. Why wasn't this happening for me? My husband watched the show with me and held me as I cried about the loss of a sacred part of our marriage. He was holding up better than me, but I could see the grief on his face and it broke my heart.

None of it made sense. If menopause is only supposed to be the end of reproductive ability then why does it result in complete ovarian failure? Why don't the ovaries continue to produce hormones—only without being fertile? Because menopause is complete ovarian failure; complete organ failure. If ovaries were *supposed* to fail at midlife, sometimes abruptly like mine did, then it would only make sense that my body would respond to this change and continue functioning as well as it had before. However instead of adapting, the body—*my* body—goes into an "ovarian hormone deficit" state. Every organ system in the body is then negatively affected, as evidenced by increased rates of cancer, heart disease and bone loss. It doesn't make sense that the amount of estrogen in the breast tissue after menopause is at about the same level as before ovarian failure. How could estrogen prevent cancer of the colon, but cause cancer of the breast? If sex drive does not change after ovarian failure then why are there so many books on sex after menopause? Why are there no books on sex after testicular failure? Is that sexist or realistic? Why does the ovary make twice as much testosterone as estrogen? I had so many questions and very few answers.

My first concern was preserving my health. If hormones were not the answer, then what was? The reports from the Women's Health Initiative confirmed that standard hormone replacement therapy is detrimental to a woman's health as she ages. If this hormone regimen didn't work then could another work? I found two small studies done on primates by the National Institutes of Health (NIH), which demonstrated that a balance of ovarian hormones could prevent or significantly reduce breast cancer.[2, 3] If this is true, where are the larger studies that would validate such an important premise? If breast cancer can be prevented in primates, studies should be done on women. If these studies show breast cancer in women can be reduced or prevented then shouldn't that be the standard of care?

I began to research how the ovaries work and why they fail so early in life. I found out that ovaries are not designed or pre-programmed to fail; rather they fail only because they are depleted of eggs. Observational studies show that the depletion of eggs can be influenced both positively and negatively. The stresses the ovaries are exposed to influence how fast or slow the eggs are used. I don't believe that my body ever expected my ovaries to fail. For a natural process, it makes more sense that ovaries would become less fertile as a woman ages, and that the ovaries would then slow down into old age and never fail. Whether a woman's body anticipates it or not, her ovaries will fail once they run out of eggs. Now that a woman's life expectancy is 80 years or more, it's up to us to try to extend ovarian function to match our extended lifetimes. Modern medicine has allowed women to choose when to have their babies. It's time for modern medicine to give women a choice about ovarian failure (menopause). Every other organ failure in the body is treated with life extending treatment, so why not the ovaries?

Women have always been told that menopause is inevitable. Together we can make menopause a choice; that is, we'll no longer have to accept menopause as inevitable. However, this can only be a reality if all of us work together toward this goal.

It's time that we change the way we think about menopause.

Key Points:
- Ovarian failure changes the way we think and feel
- Ovarian failure negatively affects the entire body
- Women now live longer than their ovaries
- The Women's Health Initiative showed that standard HRT is unhealthy
- Ovarian failure should be optional

CHAPTER 2

A COMMON LANGUAGE AND A COMMON GOAL

How we communicate shapes the way we think. In order to change the way we think we must first make sure that we're all communicating in the same way. All of us, women and our doctors, must use the same words and mean the same things. Doctors talk about female and male hormones and free and total hormone levels; drug companies talk about natural, synthetic, and bio-identical hormones; and everyone has their own personal definition of what menopause is. There are dozens of books and articles available—each with its own slightly different set of words that essentially describe the same things. Unless we all agree on the vocabulary, we'll never be able to agree upon the goal.

In order to understand the potential of ovarian function to be extended into old age, and how much healthier this would be, it's important to understand what hormones the ovaries produce and the balance created by these hormones. It's important to understand that what is currently meant by standard "hormone replacement therapy," or HRT, is very different from the balance provided by functioning ovaries. Hormone replacement therapy is a catchall phrase that is used to describe the many different ways of administering ovarian hormones in the hopes of creating a balance that is as close as possible to the balance present before menopause. Unfortunately there are no standards set, leaving individual clinicians and women to come up with their own regimens, often with disappointing results (see chapter 6 for more information).

WHAT ARE HORMONES?

Hormones are the chemical messengers of the body. The shape of a hormone, literally the shape of the molecule, determines the message that is sent. Like a lock and a key, a hormone will attach itself to a receptor with just the right shape. The strength of a hormone is determined by how well it fits into its hormone receptor. After it attaches to the receptor, the receptor then folds around the hormone to create a new shape. This new shape determines how long its effect is felt. Estradiol is a long-lasting hormone, and thus very small quantities of it are produced in the body. Progesterone is a very short-acting hormone so it is produced in much greater quantities in the body, about 100 times more than estradiol (the strongest estrogen made by the ovaries).

WHAT IS AN ESTROGEN?

Any hormone that can attach to an estrogen receptor and cause a response is called an estrogen agonist. An estrogen is considered to be either weak or strong depending on how long the response lasts and how tightly bound it is to the receptor.

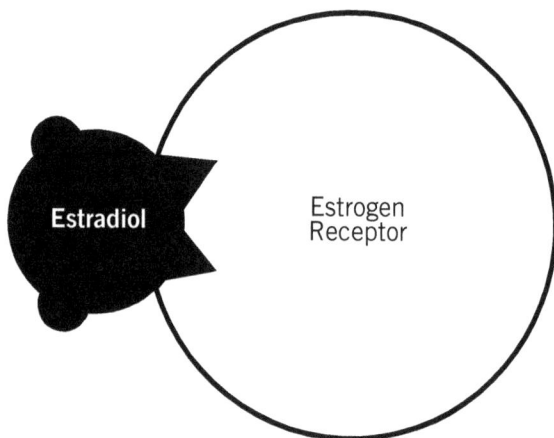

Figure 1: Estradiol with its receptor

Calling a hormone an estrogen is not descriptive of its effect on the body. For instance, Tamoxifen™ is very effective for breast cancer treatment because it is more likely to bind to estrogen receptors than the estrogen the body makes. Tamoxifen™ thus prevents the estrogen from binding to the receptor. Once Tamoxifen™ is bound to the receptor it has a very weak response, preventing the cell growth that estrogen would have stimulated. Another estrogen that is made by the body is estrone. Estrone, like Tamoxifen™, is a very weak estrogen and many times less potent than estradiol. Another estrogen is estriol. Estriol is a still weaker estrogen. Estradiol, estrone, estriol, and Tamoxifen™ are all analogs, because they attach to estrogen receptors. Each of these causes a very different response and is used for very different purposes.

HOW ESTRADIOL IS PRODUCED

Estradiol is made directly from testosterone by an enzyme called aromatase. It is made inside a developing egg within the ovary, as well as by the adrenal glands and fat tissue. First testosterone is made along the outside of the egg. From this testosterone a small amount is converted to estradiol. Then, both hormones are released into the bloodstream.[1]

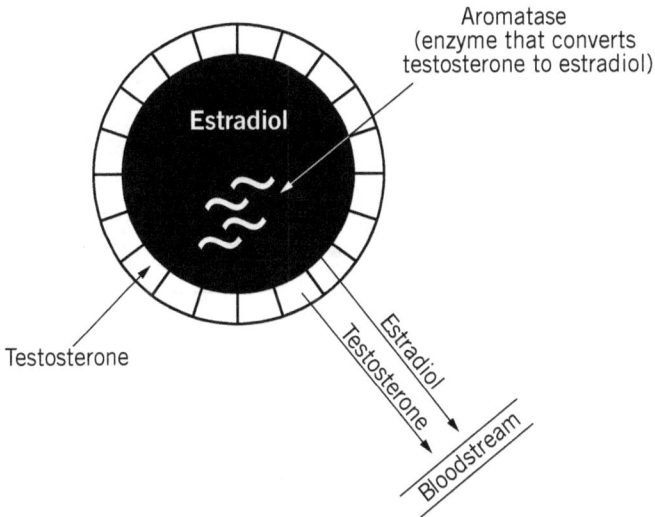

Figure 2: Hormone production in a developing egg; testosterone + aromatase (an enzyme) = estradiol

HOW ALL HORMONES ARE STORED IN THE BLOOD

In the blood, hormones are either very tightly bound to binding proteins (molecules) or unbound and "free" in the bloodstream. Hormones that are bound are not considered biologically active, which means they will not have an effect on the cells in the body. Hormones that are in a "free" or biologically active form are available for use by the body. An extremely small amount of any hormone exists in its "free" state in the blood. The "total" level of any hormone is the sum of the "free" plus the "bound" levels. Figure 3 shows the relative amounts of free and total levels of ovarian hormones. Particularly important is the extremely low percentage of free estradiol, free testosterone, and free progesterone.

Total Hormone Level = Free + Bound

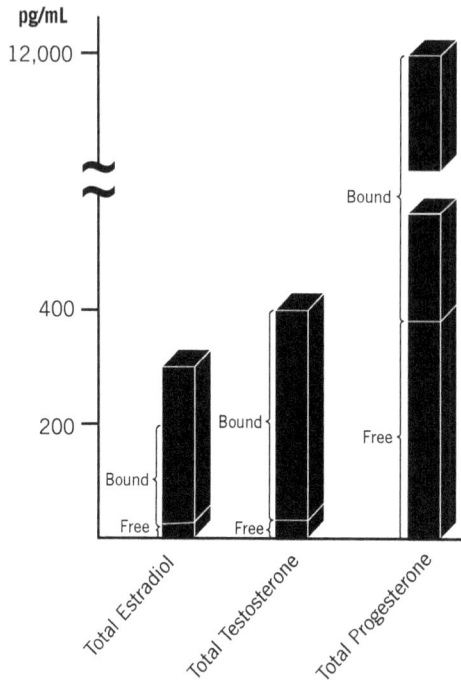

Figure 3: Free and total levels of ovarian hormones (pg/ml = picograms per milliliter)

The amount of free hormone is important, as it is the biologically active part of the hormone, the part that makes things happen. Estradiol and testosterone are bound to the same binding molecule, called sex hormone binding globulin, or SHBG for short (Figure 4). SHBG is made by the liver, and its production is affected differently by increasing levels of estradiol and testosterone. If the liver senses dramatically increasing levels of estradiol, as with an estrogen pill, it will produce more SHBG. If the liver senses dramatically increasing levels of testosterone, as with a testosterone pill, it will produce less SHBG. A slower introduction of estradiol through the skin, as with a patch, cream, or gel, will only cause a small response from the liver and the level of SHBG will go up only slightly, if at all. Similarly, a slower introduction of testosterone through the skin, as with a patch, cream, or gel, will only cause a small response from the liver and the level of SHBG will only go down slightly, if at all. Another important benefit of using the transdermal method is that the hormones are absorbed directly into the skin, bypassing the liver. Also, transdermal application of estrogen and testosterone does not increase triglyceride levels, which is a risk factor for heart disease. The level of SHBG is very important because higher levels decrease the amount of free estradiol and free testosterone hormone in the blood.

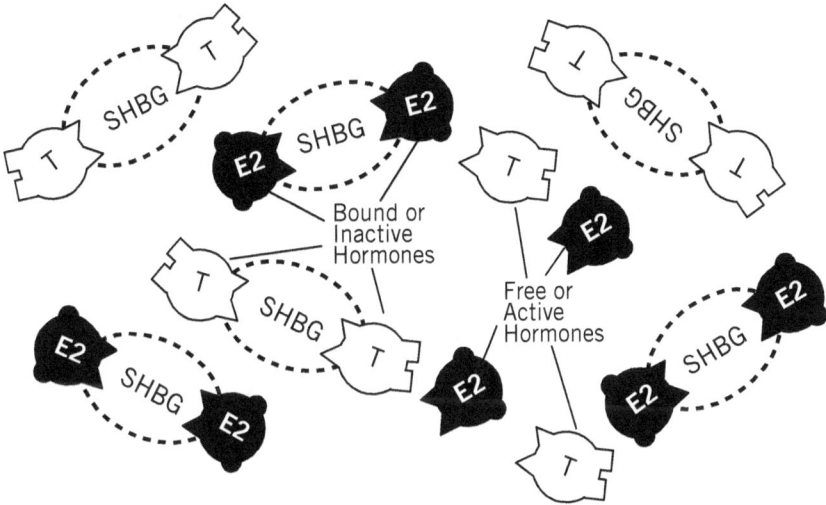

Figure 4: Higher levels of SHBG means less free estradiol and free testosterone

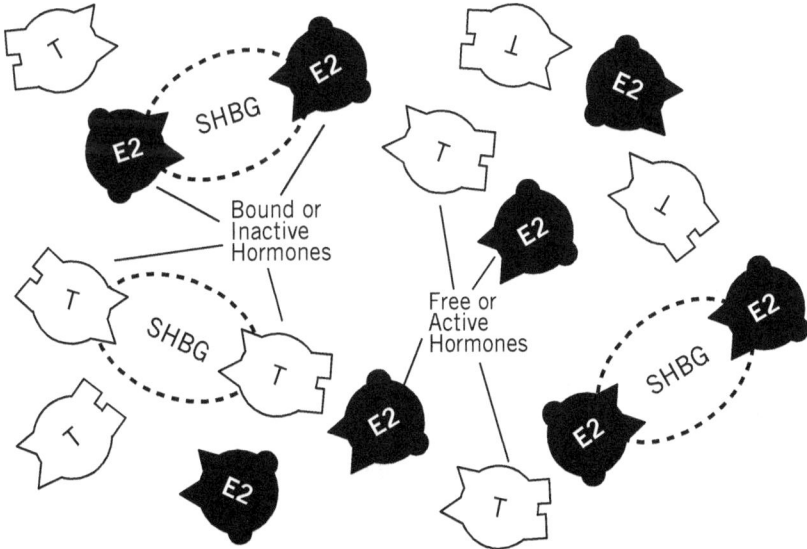

Figure 5: Less SHBG means higher levels of free estradiol and free testosterone

HORMONAL PRODUCTS

To prevent menopause or to re-establish an ovarian hormone balance, hormonal products that contain estradiol, testosterone, or progesterone or some combination of these hormones would be necessary. To better understand treatment related to ovarian health it is important that everyone use the same name for the same product. Below is a list of common names for different ovarian hormones.

Estradiol is called:
1) Estradiol
2) 17beta-Estradiol
3) 17-Estradiol
4) E2
5) Estradiol USP
6) Estrogen

Testosterone is called:
1) Testosterone
2) T
3) Testosterone USP

Progesterone is called:
1) Progesterone
2) P4
3) Progesterone USP

WHAT IS THE DIFFERENCE BETWEEN SYNTHETIC, NATURAL AND PATENTED HORMONES?

Hormones are often marketed as natural, which makes them sound like they are better than synthetic hormones. It is not enough to call a hormone product natural or synthetic to know what to expect from it. What makes a hormone effective is its chemical structure, not its source. The most effective are bio-identical hormones, which are exact copies of the hormones that your body naturally produces and uses. With the exception of a few hormone preparations that are derived from urine (Figure 6), all bio-identical hormones are manufactured in a laboratory, often from a plant source. What

28

is important is to use hormones that are bio-identical and in the appropriate doses to the ones your body naturally produces to get as close to the same effect as possible. Bio-identical hormones are exact copies of the hormones the body manufactures, only made in a laboratory, so new and different side effects would be minimal, if any.

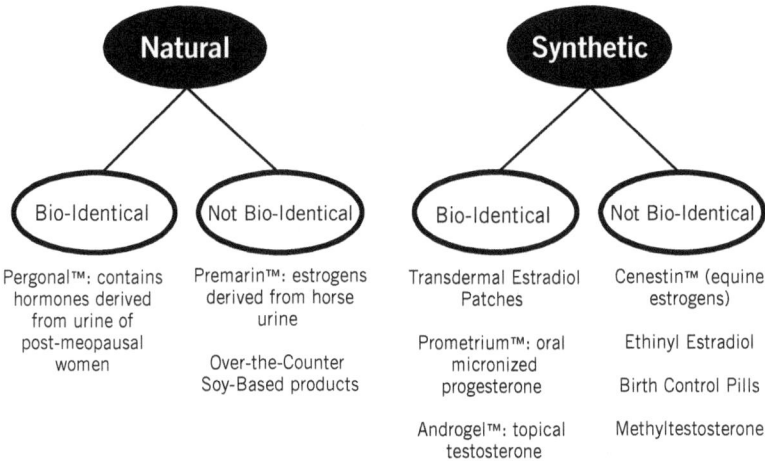

Figure 6: Examples of natural, synthetic and patented hormones

Pharmaceutical companies know this. They start with a bio-identical hormone, one that has the same molecular structure of a hormone the body naturally produces. They then change it as little as possible, but just enough to get a patent on it. The resulting hormone is subsequently used in place of the bio-identical hormone. The effect of this new hormone is similar but not the same as the original hormone and usually has side effects, because it is a hormone the body does not naturally produce. Pharmaceutical companies can make much more money by selling patented hormones rather than non-patented hormones. This is because patented hormones cannot be sold by any other company, nor can generic versions be made by any other company, for seventeen years. This monopoly allows companies to make more money from patented hormones. Bio-identical hormones cannot be patented; the only thing that *can* be patented is the process by which these hormones are manufactured. This significantly limits their profit potential.

WHY SAY OVARIAN FAILURE INSTEAD OF MENOPAUSE?

The word menopause is from a Greek phrase that means "the end month to cease to come." So, the word menopause actually means the last month ovarian function occurred, which would mean your very last period. Thus the word menopause does not describe ovarian function. Instead, it describes ovarian failure. The word peri-menopause has come to mean either: a) the time when menstrual cycles have become irregular; or b) symptoms of impending ovarian failure are observed.

The terms menopause and peri-menopause can be used in a variety of ways, all with different meanings. I think it's clearer and more understandable to say *ovarian failure* and *failing ovaries*. These terms may seem harsh, but they're actually much closer to truth. It's more likely that we'll be able to understand each other—and that our doctors will understand the gravity of our situations—if we speak of failing ovaries rather than peri-menopause. The use of such direct language will also encourage all of us to make clearer, wiser decisions for ourselves.

Some women have their ovaries removed surgically and some women take medications that harm their ovaries so that they no longer function. These women have all the same symptoms as women with ovarian failure; the symptoms just occur more abruptly. Another term for menopause caused by surgical removal of the ovaries is surgical castration or surgical menopause. And another term for ovaries that have failed due to medication, like chemotherapy, is chemical castration. Hormone levels after menopause and castration are the same. Indeed the effect of menopause, no matter the cause, is the same as castration.

Whether ovarian failure is a result of injury, surgery, medication or an organ failing on its own, it's still castration. Every woman who outlives her ovaries is living out her life castrated. The thought of all men over age 50 being castrated is overwhelming harsh. Yet somehow the idea of all women living out their lives castrated is not only palatable, but also encouraged by the medical profession. Women are told that this is their lot in life. There has never been a real attempt by the medical profession to replace ovarian function with ovarian hormones. Although the Women's Health Initiative's goal was to "investigate strategies to prevent and control common causes of morbidity and mortality"[2] such as heart disease, bone loss, and cancer, it was presented as hormone replacement therapy (HRT) to attract participants. This makes it sound like it replaces the function of the ovaries. Yet a comparison of HRT to pre-menopausal levels of ovarian hormones shows that HRT is not based on ovarian function at all. It contains only minimal amounts of normal ovarian hormones, and was never intended to replace ovarian function (see chapter 6 for more information).

Doctors, both female and male, tell women that being menopausal is normal and natural, which is the equivalent of saying that being castrated is normal and natural. They counsel women to find a way to live with it and still function as if they weren't castrated. It's time for us to be honest with ourselves, and for our doctors to be honest with us. Let's finally acknowledge menopause for what it is and what it isn't.

OVARIAN HORMONES HAVE MULTIPLE FUNCTIONS

Every organ system in the body uses the primary ovarian hormones— testosterone, progesterone and estradiol—to function; therefore ovarian failure affects every organ in the body. The ovaries make a major contribution to maintaining the health of a woman beyond simply providing eggs for reproduction, and estradiol and testosterone for sex drive. Estradiol has long been referred to as the female hormone; and testosterone, as the male hormone. But there really is no such thing as a male or female hormone. Men and women simply make different amounts of the same hormones.

One way to demonstrate how many organ systems ovarian hormones influence is to look at where estrogen, androgen and progesterone receptors are located throughout the body. Below is a partial list of different areas of the body that depend on ovarian hormones for optimal functioning, and what happens to these organs when the ovaries fail.

Organ System	After Ovarian Failure
Breast	30-fold increase in breast cancer[3], reduction in fat in breasts, which causes them to shrink and sag, loss of sensitivity and erection in nipples
Blood Vessels, Heart	Accelerated stiffness of the arteries[4], increase in blood pressure, significant increased risk of heart disease[5], heart palpitations[6], hot flashes

31

Organ System	After Ovarian Failure
Mouth, Teeth	Dry mouth, increase in periodontal disease, increased risk of tooth loss from osteoporosis, abnormal taste sensation, menopausal gingivostomatitis, shrinking gums, increase in dental caries (cavities)[7, 8]
Skin	Accelerated degenerative changes, lose of elasticity, increase in wrinkles, dry skin[3], loss of sensitivity to touch, tingling in hands and feet
Brain	"Foggy" thinking, memory problems[10]
Uterus	15-fold increase in uterine cancer after ovarian failure[3]
Vagina, Clitoris	Lost elasticity and shrinkage (which can make intercourse very painful), increased risk of tear in vaginal lining, significant loss of clitoral sensitivity, significantly decreased sexual response (arousal and orgasm),[11, 12] anorgasmia (inability to achieve orgasm)[12]
Esophagus	Increase in heartburn
Gastrointestinal Tract	Increased gas, bloating, flatulence[13] in 2/3 of women
Liver	Increase in cholesterol and other lipids
Bone	Bone loss for every woman, to varying degrees; osteoporosis is also a risk factor for gum disease,[14] increased joint pain/ache
Eyes, Ears	Increased prevalence in dry eye, ringing in the ears (tinnitus), dizziness
Bladder, Urethra	Shrinking bladder and urethra, increased urine leakage, more frequent urination
Metabolism Fat Distribution	Weight gain, slower metabolism,[15] hypothyroidism, redistribution of fat to abdomen,[16] decreasing insulin sensitivity
Muscle	Decreased muscle tone and strength[17, 18]
Sleep	Insomnia in 50 % of women over 50, increased prevalence of sleep disorder breathing (sleep apnea),[19, 20] increase in snoring[21]
Hair, Nails	Head hair loss, thinning of pubic hair, increased facial hair, brittle fingernails
Nervous System	Anxiety, mood swings, depression

Table 1: How ovarian failure affects the organs in the body

Every organ system in the body uses ovarian hormones to function. It follows then that ovarian failure negatively affects every organ in the body.

In addition to the three types of hormones normally associated with the ovaries, estrogen, androgen and progesterone, there are many others. The ovaries also produce hormones that communicate with the brain. And, they make different hormones in the first part of the menstrual cycle, before ovulation, than they do in the second part of the cycle, after ovulation. Several small studies have shown that women who have breast cancer surgery in the second part of their menstrual cycle have a slightly higher survival rate than those who have surgery in the first part of their menstrual cycle.[22, 23] This may have to do with the presence of progesterone. It also may be a result of the kind of hormones produced in the second part of the menstrual cycle. These kinds of studies raise interesting questions and hopefully, with more of them undertaken in the future, we'll have more answers.

Another example of the impact functioning ovaries have on the whole body can be seen in the way ovarian hormones may protect women from heart disease. As ovaries begin to fail, they produce less and less ovarian hormones until, after ovarian failure, production ceases completely. Studies have shown that at the same time that levels of hormones go down, arterial plaque formation goes up.[24,25,26] It's interesting to note that while the testes also make the same hormones, they do make less than the ovaries. This suggests that a *lack* of ovarian hormones may contribute to the development of heart disease, and may explain why men get heart disease about 10 years earlier, on average, than women. Again, only more studies can give us the answers that we're looking for.

Preventing menopause means preventing ovarian failure. To do this we must work together, speak the same language and share the same goals. We need to understand what we're doing, and why. The ovaries are underappreciated organs. They contribute a great deal to a woman's overall sense of well-being, and thus treatment should be offered to help ovaries function for as long as possible. Menopause is as harsh as castration because it's the same as castration. We must do what we can to make the present generation the last to suffer ovarian failure, and make menopause optional.

Key Points:

- All of us, doctors and women, need to speak the same language to achieve the goal of preventing ovarian failure
- Most hormones in the blood are inactive, or "bound up"
- Only the "free" part of the total hormone level has an effect on the cells in the body
- Given a choice, go with bio-identical hormones
- Hormone levels and ratios are very different before and after ovarian failure
- Ovarian hormones, estrogen, androgen, and progesterone, positively affect the entire body, and their loss may be a key reason why there is an acceleration of heart disease as ovaries fail.
- Menopause is ovarian failure

CHAPTER 3

WHY PREVENT OVARIAN
FAILURE?

Our goal is to prevent ovarian failure, but what does that mean, and why is it our goal? What are the benefits of extending ovarian function for an additional 20 to 30 years? If experiencing ovarian failure around age 50 has been the norm for thousands of years, why is it a problem now? Look at the advertisements for drugs that treat the results of ovarian failure, such as heart disease and osteoporosis. Look at the change in cancer risk after ovarian failure. Any of these risks would be reason enough. Taken together, they are a clear indication of the need to prevent ovarian failure.

WHAT IS OVARIAN FAILURE?
Ovarian failure means that the ovaries have failed and are no longer producing hormones. Ovarian failure is the same thing as menopause. Any estrogen, testosterone or progesterone in the body after ovarian failure is largely produced by the adrenal glands and fat deposits in the body. For this reason, women who are heavier have slightly higher levels of hormones. However, the level of each hormone is a fraction of what was once produced by the ovaries (see Figure 7). Before ovarian failure the level of testosterone is about 2–3 times higher than estradiol, and progesterone is about 100 times higher. After ovarian failure the level of testosterone is about 10–20 times higher than estradiol, and progesterone is about 40 times higher. After ovarian failure a very small amount of estradiol, testosterone and progesterone is made by the adrenal gland. The level of estradiol is about 25 times less, testosterone is about half, and progesterone is about 40 times less.

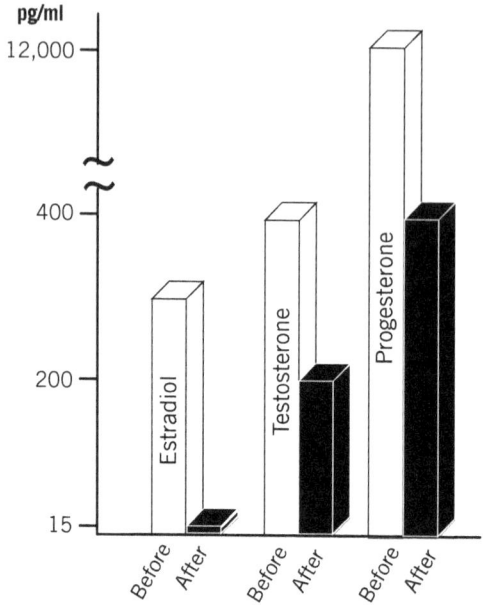

Figure 7: Levels of ovarian hormones before and after ovarian failure

IS OVARIAN FAILURE NATURAL, NORMAL OR NEITHER?

Women typically experience a very fertile time in early adulthood and then decreasing fertility as they age. Approaching 40 years old a woman experiences significantly reduced fertility, even though her ovaries continue to function (see Figure 8).

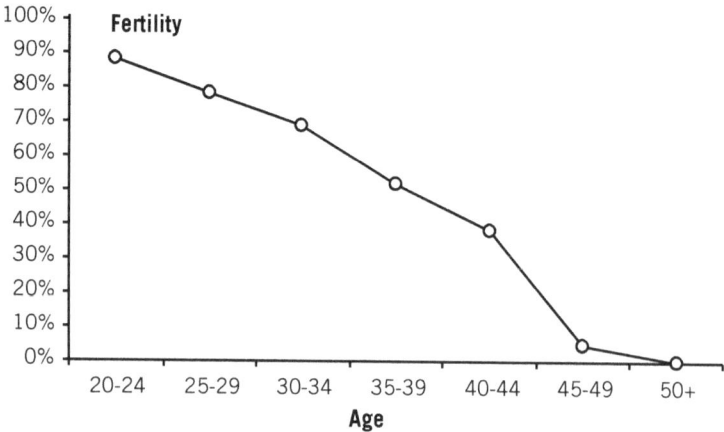

Figure 8: Fertility vs. age

36

Having fewer children later in life ensures that greater resources are available for raising the children we have in our youth.[1] But ovarian failure is not healthy for a woman who can expect to live for more than 80 years. Ovarian failure has no health benefits, nor does the body adapt to the loss of ovarian function. In fact, quite the opposite is true.

One of the most startling findings from my research is that once the ovaries fail and stop producing estradiol, the breast (as well as other areas of the body) continues to convert testosterone into estradiol, and as a woman ages the rate of production increases.[2] By converting testosterone into estradiol, the breast retains levels of estradiol that are similar to pre-ovarian failure levels. Testosterone keeps the growth of breast tissue in check, and with the reduction in testosterone that is a result of ovarian failure, the breasts become a prime target for cancer. In other words, the conversion of testosterone into estradiol by the breast tissue may at least in part explain the dramatic and alarming increase in breast cancer rates after ovarian failure. (Breast cancer is actually quite rare in women with ovarian function.) The female body was designed to function well with ovarian function, not without.

Women in the last hundred years are the first in history to live a substantial part of their lives with ovarian failure. Before that time, it was rare for a woman to live past 50; so most women did not experience ovarian failure during their lifetimes. Women now suffer ovarian failure in mid-life. Mid-life to us means the mid-forties to mid-fifties. A hundred years ago midlife meant age 20 to 25, wherein the highest level of fertility was experienced. Age 45 to 55 meant end of life and very low fertility (see Figure 8).[3] Now, almost everyone, men and women, lives past the age of 50. The average life span has been extended to more than 80 years. Current ovarian function, however, may have evolved for a shorter life span. Understanding how the ovary works and how eggs are recruited and matured can make it possible to *extend* the function of the ovaries another 20 to 30 years, thus eliminating early depletion of the ovaries and ovarian failure.

The breasts are not the only organs to suffer. Many organ systems would benefit from continued ovarian function. Breast cancer would become rare, as it is in women with ovarian function. Heart disease would be delayed or prevented. And, preventing ovarian failure by extending the life of the ovaries, or by continuing to foster a balance of ovarian hormones after ovarian failure has occurred, means that a woman's body wouldn't suffer the ravages of an ovarian hormone deficient state.

Currently, ovarian failure is referred to as an "estrogen deficient state"—and the effects of estrogen deficiency are well documented. While the ovaries produce about one-third of the androgens in a woman's body, the effects of a reduction in androgens are not as well defined. After ovarian failure women are at risk of "female androgen insufficiency." The symptoms for this include low libido, decreased energy, and loss of feelings of well-being. Discussion with your doctor can help you figure out if female androgen insufficiency is a problem for you.[4]

Women's bodies make about 71 percent of the androgens that men's bodies make, which would suggest that androgens play an important role in their overall functioning.[5] There are many different types of androgens, testosterone being just one. Approximately one-third of the androgens in a woman's body come from her ovaries; one-third from fat stores on her body; and one-third from her adrenal glands, which are small organs that sit on top of the kidneys (see Figure 9).

Testosterone Production

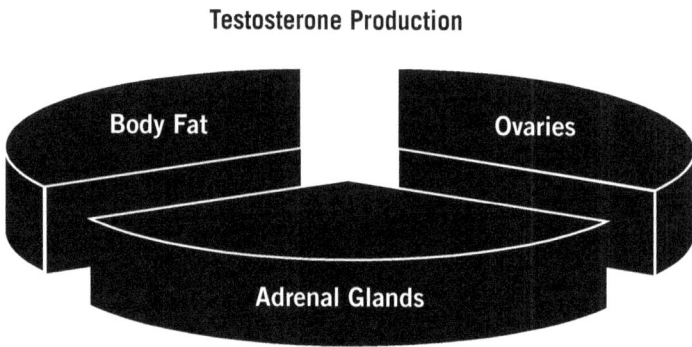

Figure 9: Androgen production in women (1/3 from ovaries; 1/3 from body fat; and 1/3 from adrenal glands)

Like every other organ, ovaries are important to the healthy functioning of a woman's entire body. As the ovaries begin to fail, risk factors for heart disease begin to increase, as does risk of breast cancer. Sexual response begins to decline, risk factors for osteoporosis begin to increase, and fertility begins to drop. Every organ system in the body thus responds negatively to the failure of the ovaries (see Table 1).

Ovarian failure is just what happens when the ovaries run out of eggs. The body doesn't plan for the ovaries to fail at any particular age. Rather, ovaries function well for high fertility in a woman's youth, and low fertility near the end of a woman's life. Now that our lives have been extended by an average of 30 years, we must urge our doctors to help our ovaries catch up—so they too can last a lifetime. Women's bodies were never meant to live without all of their organs.

HOW BREAST TISSUE RESPONDS TO OVARIAN FAILURE

The breast responds differently to ovarian failure than do other organs in the body. As we've already discussed, the breasts attempt to adapt to the low levels of estradiol, also known as "estradiol starvation." Something has to happen in the breast to restore estradiol levels to pre-ovarian failure levels. The same enzyme that converts testosterone to estradiol in the egg, aromatase, which is also in the bones, fat, liver, brain and breast tissue, becomes four to five times more sensitive in breast tissue. The increased sensitivity of the aromatase enzyme is able to convert enough testosterone into estradiol to bring the estradiol level within the breast tissue up to pre-ovarian failure levels, while testosterone and progesterone levels remain in the ovarian failure range. And yet as you'll see, testosterone is important to the prevention of breast cancer.

HOW TESTOSTERONE MAY PROTECT AGAINST BREAST CANCER

Testosterone may protect breast tissue because of how it acts upon the estrogen receptors in the breast. Two types of estrogen receptors have been found. They are called Estrogen Receptor alpha (ER alpha) and Estrogen Receptor beta (ER beta). The ratio of these two receptors may play an important role in the development of breast cancer. This ratio appears to indicate how invasive a breast cancer may be. Estradiol is known to increase ER alpha; while testosterone has been shown to decrease ER alpha and increase ER beta. Prior to ovarian failure, there is a greater amount of ER beta than there is ER alpha. After ovarian failure this is reversed, so that there is a greater amount of ER alpha than there is ER beta (see Figure 10). This shift in the ratio of estrogen receptors is a direct result of continually declining testosterone levels as ovaries fail.[6,7,8,9,10,11] This raises the question of whether maintaining pre-menopausal levels of estradiol and testosterone would result in a lower risk of breast cancer.

Ovarian Function	Ovarian Failure
ER Alpha / ER Beta	ER Alpha / ER Beta
Risk of Breast Cancer: 1 woman in 2200	Risk of Breast Cancer: 1 woman in 10

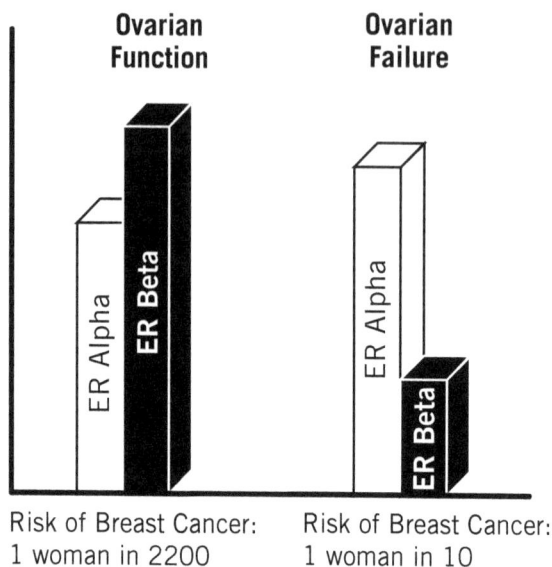

Figure 10: Ratio of estrogen receptors before and after ovarian failure

STUDIES CLEARLY DEMONSTRATE HOW TESTOSTERONE PREVENTS BREAST CANCER

Knowing that testosterone can decrease ER alpha and increase ER beta, the National Institutes of Health (NIH) sponsored two studies (in 2000 and 2002) on primates. Both studies were designed to investigate testosterone's ability to reverse the cell growth (proliferation) caused by the ER alpha dominance seen in women with ovarian failure, and also to see if a cancer gene, MYC, would be suppressed. The results were consistent. The conclusion from the study undertaken in 2000 was as follows:

> "In summary, the present data show that addition of androgen to estrogen treatment reduces mammary epithelial proliferation and ER expression, suggesting that androgens may protect against breast cancer, by analogy with progesterone's protective effects on the uterus."[11]

And the conclusion from the study undertaken in 2002:

> "In summary, the present data show that androgens reduce mammary epithelial proliferation and regulate mammary epithelial ER alpha and ER beta and MYC expression, suggesting that androgens

40

may protect against breast cancer, by analogy with progesterone's protective effects upon the uterus. These considerations suggest that physiological estrogen/androgen "replacement" therapy may be beneficial to girls and women with ovarian failure."[8]

Even though these studies were done on primates, the significance of these findings cannot be overstated. The levels of estradiol used in both studies were the same as those normally found in women with ovarian function, and were 15 to 25 times the levels found in women with ovarian failure. The modest amount of total testosterone used in these experiments was in the mid-normal range of adult women with ovarian function (40 ng/dL), and completely reversed the growth of cells caused by estradiol alone.

A balance of estradiol and testosterone in the normal adult range creates a balance of ER alpha and ER beta receptors that decreases the expression of the MYC gene. This may contribute to the prevention of breast cancer. Estradiol alone increased expression of ER alpha, which in turn stimulated MYC expression, which in turn increased the risk of breast cancer. These studies on primates suggest that either continuing ovarian function or restoring normal ovarian hormonal balance to women with ovarian failure may have a significant impact on preventing breast cancer.

BREAST CANCER AND HYPOGONADISM

Being hypogonadal, for a man or a woman, means having abnormally low levels of the sex hormones estradiol, testosterone, and progesterone. Ovarian failure is a hypogonadal state, as is testicular failure. Breast cancer is a disease that usually strikes hypogonadal women. Approximately 80 percent of women diagnosed with breast cancer are hypogonadal.

The most frequently diagnosed type of breast cancer in women after ovarian failure is the same as that diagnosed in men: estrogen receptor positive breast cancer, or ER+. This type of breast cancer is associated with hypogonadism in women (ovarian failure). Breast cancer in men accounts for about 1 percent of all breast cancers. It is similar to breast cancer in women however, and is managed and treated similarly.[12, 13] A man's lifetime exposure to estradiol is about half of a women's lifetime exposure. Men have much higher levels of total estradiol than women with ovarian failure. Even so, men still have a significantly lower risk of breast cancer.

Men have a total estradiol level of 25-50 pg/ml; while women with ovarian failure have a total estradiol level of 12-20 pg/ml.[14, 15] This means that men have *2 to 3 times* the level of total estradiol than women with ovarian failure. Even though women have less estradiol in their breast tissue than men, breast cancer is diagnosed in 100 women for every 1 man with the disease. The incidence of male breast cancer is so low that it is one of the rarest of all malignancies, occurring in just 0.07 percent of men.

While there are many therapies that are being explored to treat and potentially cure breast cancer, none involve maintaining ovarian function to help keep the breasts healthy. This kind of research deserves focus because it not only has the potential to prevent breast cancer, but also to help maintain the quality of life for women as they age.

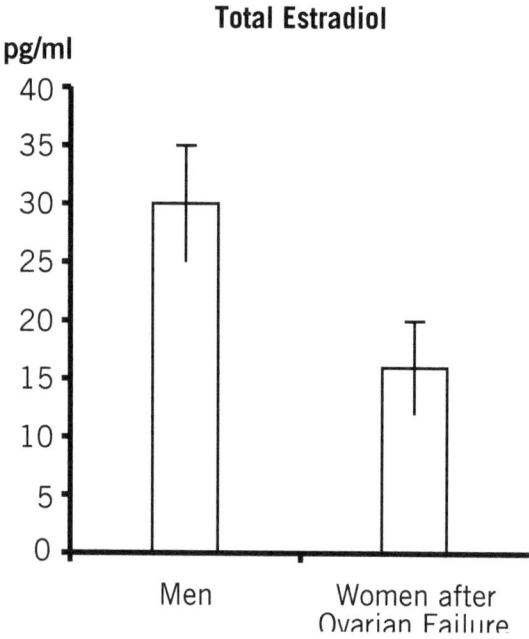

Figure 11: Total estradiol for men and women after ovarian failure

RISK OF CANCER AND OVARIAN FAILURE

Of all the organs in the body, the breasts suffer the biggest increase in cancer and would have the greatest reduction in cancer rates if ovarian function were extended into old age. Before ovarian failure breast cancer is very rare. At age

42

25, 1 in 20,000 women will be diagnosed with breast cancer. As women get older that risk steadily increases, until by age 80 the risk is 1 in 9.[16] Breast cancer is extremely rare when ovarian hormone levels are at their highest, and the risk is highest when levels are at their lowest. This would suggest that a balance of ovarian hormones plays an important role in maintaining a healthy hormonal balance within the breast.

Uterine cancer rates also go up after ovarian failure, but not as dramatically as breast cancer rates. Uterine cancer increases from about 1 in 200 to 1 in 37 over a woman's lifetime. Rates of ovarian cancer, however, are very low over the course of a woman's lifetime. Ovarian cancer rates only go up slightly after ovarian failure. Uterine and ovarian cancers also show an unhealthy disruption in the ratio of estrogen receptors alpha and beta; however, not to the extent that the breast does[17]. This disruption may also lead to an increase in the expression of the MYC gene.

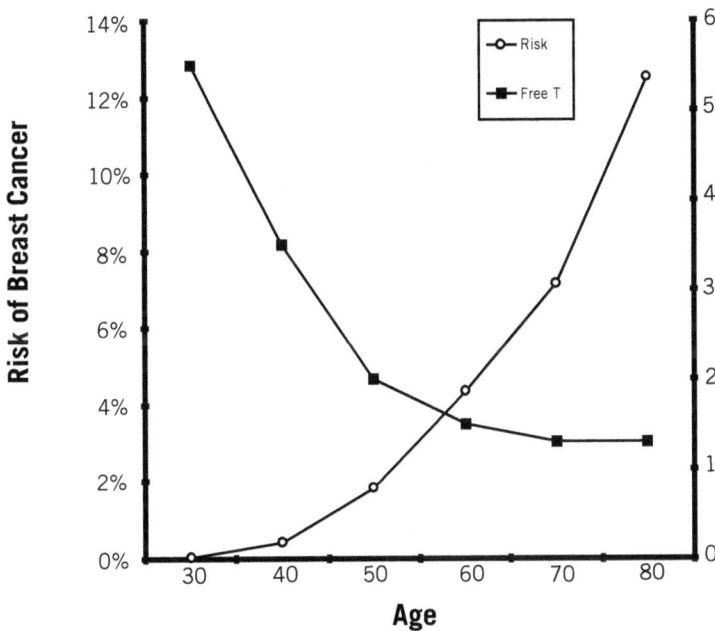

Figure 12: Breast cancer rates by age

43

Like breast cancer, uterine cancer and ovarian cancer primarily stem from an over expression of the MYC gene and its relationship to estrogen receptors alpha and beta.[18, 19, 20] Testosterone is one of the regulators of the MYC gene and suppresses its expression. Therefore, as testosterone levels fall, the incidence of these cancers goes up. The female genital system loses an important protection from cancer when the ovaries fail. Figure 12 clearly shows a dramatic rise in breast cancer as free testosterone levels fall.

HOW OVARIAN FAILURE AFFECTS YOUR RISK OF HEART DISEASE

Heart disease is rare in women under age 45. Heart disease, also called coronary artery disease (CAD), occurs when a build-up of fatty deposits or plaque begins to form along the lining of the blood vessels. As ovarian function declines, the risk of heart disease rises dramatically. Women with ovarian failure who are under the age of 40 experience this increased risk of heart disease even sooner. Many more women die of heart disease than breast cancer. One of every two women will die of heart disease, compared to 1 of 25 for breast cancer (see "Ovarian Hormones Have Multiple Functions" on page 31).[21]

We know that high cholesterol, high triglycerides, and high LDL levels are unhealthy. However there *is* one level that we want to be high, and that's HDL, or high density lipoprotein. A high HDL level is considered a good thing, as HDL promotes heart health by preventing heart disease. The higher a woman's level of HDL, the lower her risk of heart disease. HDL helps to prevent heart disease by transporting cholesterol away from places where it can be deposited, like blood vessels. It brings it to the liver to be processed and excreted from the body.

In general, young women have a higher HDL than men. After ovarian failure 20 percent of women continue to have desirable levels of HDL, which is supposed to help protect them from heart disease. Unfortunately, for that 20 percent of women, a higher level of HDL is no longer as protective after ovarian failure, even for those who exercise,[22] and the risk of heart disease becomes the same as, or greater than, a man's. Why does this occur?

For both women and men, HDL protects the heart in at least two ways. It is well documented that HDL carries cholesterol from the blood to the liver, which can help reduce or delay plaque formation in the arteries. A study published in *The Journal of Clinical Investigation* in May 2003 showed that another potential benefit of HDL is how it works together with estradiol.[23]

Estradiol can be a component of HDL in the blood, and this HDL can deliver the estradiol to the blood vessels to produce an enzyme, nitric oxide synthase, or NOS. NOS in turn helps make nitric oxide (NO). NO is very important to the health of the vascular system. It increases the relaxation of the blood vessels. Blood vessels that are more relaxed are healthier than when they're stiff. This study looked at how HDL and estradiol work together in women before and after ovarian failure, and in men. The findings are very important because they provide additional insight into why women are still at increased risk of heart disease, even with desirable levels of HDL, after ovarian failure. The study showed an additional benefit of HDL, beyond its ability to help take cholesterol out of the blood. It showed that:

1) Women with ovarian function had adequate nitric oxide production.
2) Men had nitric oxide production, but not nearly as much as women with ovarian function.
3) After ovarian failure, women had production rates of nitric oxide that were lower than those found in men.

To confirm that the lack of estradiol was the reason for such a low response in women with ovarian failure, the experiment was run again. This time it was run with women who had ovarian failure and were given estradiol, and the women who were given estradiol produced higher levels of NO. The results were dose dependent; meaning that as estradiol levels increased, so did levels of NO.[24, 25] As noted above, the higher levels of NO lead to healthier, more relaxed blood vessels.

Another important benefit of higher NO levels and more relaxed blood vessels is prevention of high blood pressure. After ovarian failure, blood pressure goes up in every woman. The increase in blood pressure from a loss of ovarian function may be minimal. However it occurs in every woman who has abnormally low levels of estradiol.[26, 27] Extending ovarian function into old age would have a significant positive effect on levels of NO and heart health.

OVARIAN FUNCTION AND HEART DISEASE

It has long been accepted that women are vulnerable to heart disease as they age because their estradiol levels drop after their ovaries fail. It is generally believed that prior to ovarian failure, women's higher levels of estradiol completely protected them from heart disease by keeping their lipid levels low. However, a series of interesting papers has been written documenting that this does not in fact occur.[28] One of these papers includes an important study that was published in the *Journal of Human Reproduction* in August 2003,[29] which redirected the focus on risk factors for heart disease from a lack of estradiol, to overall declining ovarian function.

This study looked at risk factors for heart disease in women who had slightly elevated estradiol levels (as estradiol levels actually go up slightly about 10 years before the ovaries fail). It was expected that an increase in estradiol would keep risk factors for heart disease low; however, this is not what was discovered. Instead, as levels of FSH (follicle stimulating hormone) and estradiol rose, so did the risk factors for heart disease—every one of them. Levels of LDL, triglycerides, and total cholesterol increased slightly, but so, fortunately, did HDL. So what does this mean? Well, the study demonstrated that estradiol alone is not enough to maintain healthy lipid levels. It highlighted the fact that a change in ovarian function and not just a loss of estradiol was responsible for increasing lipid levels.

It could be that there are other products that are produced by the ovaries that have yet to be discovered, or are underappreciated (see "Ovarian Hormones Have Multiple Functions" on page 31). One thing *is* clear: ovarian function protects women from heart disease, and ovarian failure does not.

OSTEOPOROSIS

With continued ovarian function into old age osteoporosis would become as rare as it is before age 40. Estradiol and testosterone together—not just estradiol alone—contribute to strong bones. Osteoporosis occurs because levels of estradiol and testosterone have fallen below the minimum required to maintain bone density. Remember, if estradiol is replaced with an estradiol pill, the binding hormone for estradiol and testosterone is doubled, which significantly lowers the free levels of testosterone. If estradiol is taken in through the skin then the levels of testosterone would remain virtually unchanged (see Table 5). The minimum levels needed to maintain bone density are 18 pg/ml of total estradiol, and 6.0 pg/ml of free testosterone. After ovarian failure, total estradiol levels are typically between 12–20 pg/ml, and free testosterone is 1.7 pg/ml (see Table 2). This puts every woman living with ovarian failure at risk for bone loss and osteoporosis.

SLEEP

As ovaries begin to fail and progesterone levels begin to fluctuate, about 40 percent of women will experience trouble falling and staying asleep. By age 50 about 50 percent of women continue to have trouble in this respect, and an increase is seen in sleep apnea. According to the National Sleep Foundation, "Sleep apnea is a serious sleep disorder that is characterized by snoring, interrupted breathing during sleep or excessive daytime sleepiness. Recent studies have also found that sleep apnea is associated with increased blood pressure, a risk for cardiovascular disease and stroke."[30]

Can this change in sleep patterns be due to a drop in melatonin, or a drop in the hormones produced by the ovaries? Actually, the answer is both—melatonin and ovarian hormones work together. Some studies have shown that as estradiol levels fall, production of melatonin increases. This suggests that more melatonin would make it easier to fall and stay asleep. However, this is not necessarily what happens. Some women can fall but not stay asleep for a whole night. Others find it difficult both to fall and stay asleep. Taking a melatonin supplement has been shown to help a person fall asleep but not stay asleep.[31] What does make a difference is replacing the progesterone and estradiol lost when the ovaries fail. When progesterone and estradiol are replaced, it is often easier both to fall asleep and stay asleep. Progesterone and estradiol together are an effective treatment for sleep troubles related to failing ovaries. It is worth noting too that in studies comparing the effectiveness of different types of progesterone to improve sleep quality, it is the bio-identical version of progesterone that is most effective.[32]

HOW OVARIAN HORMONES AND MELATONIN WORK TOGETHER

There is a special area in the brain that is responsible for helping a person fall and stay asleep. This area is very sensitive to changes in the levels of nitric oxide. Recall that nitric oxide (NO) is a powerful substance that can help the blood vessels to relax. Nitric oxide helps to regulate when a person sleeps and wakes up, and thus changes in the levels of NO may disrupt sleep.[33] Melatonin is also important in how well a person sleeps. Sometimes levels of melatonin decrease as a person gets older. While this decrease may be thought to be the cause of the sleep disruption, the first signs often occur at the time ovaries begin to fail and progesterone levels drop or fluctuate.[34] So it is unlikely that a decrease in melatonin is solely to blame for a change in sleep patterns.

A study undertaken in Italy highlights how estradiol and melatonin work together to increase the level of nitric oxide.[35] In this study melatonin levels in women living with ovarian failure were measured. Levels of nitric oxide were also measured. Women with similar levels of melatonin and nitric oxide were separated into two groups. Each group was given a melatonin supplement, which substantially raised their melatonin levels. One group was then given an estradiol patch; and the other group a placebo. All participants had their levels of nitric oxide checked. The women who received the estradiol patch had a measurable increase in their levels of nitric oxide, while the women who were taking a placebo had no change. Based on results of the study the authors concluded that without adequate levels of estradiol, the added melatonin was completely ineffective.

This is important information for women to have. There are many variables that influence sleep. However, two of these important variables can be addressed: melatonin levels and estradiol levels. Having normal levels of both significantly impacts the ability to fall and stay asleep. It is now easier, however, to see why some women suffer sleep problems around the time their ovaries begin to fail. The loss of estradiol from ovarian failure is followed by a decline in production of nitric oxide, which is followed by disruption in sleep. Therefore maintaining ovarian function or ovarian hormonal balance would likely reduce sleep disruptions.

WEIGHT GAIN AND MUSCLE TONE

Something all women share as their ovaries fail is weight gain, particularly around the abdomen. For some the gain is a few pounds, while others gain more than they ever thought they would. Extra weight gain, especially around the mid-section, is associated with an increased risk of heart disease and diabetes. As ovaries begin to fail and ovarian hormone production decreases, women begin to put on weight. One of the reasons women put on weight is because their metabolism slows in response to a decrease in muscle mass. Less ovarian hormones, particularly testosterone, means less muscle mass and a slower metabolism. If a woman continues to eat as she always has, and expends less energy, then the extra energy she no longer burns is stored as fat.[36]

Unfortunately, the fat goes straight to the abdomen.[37] The reason weight accumulates around the middle is directly related to the hormone cortisol, and the enzymes that influence how much of it is metabolized. As ovaries begin to fail and the estrogen levels begin to change, the amount of enzymes in the fat around the abdomen also changes. The result of decreasing estradiol levels is that extra calories are more easily stored as fat around the abdomen, instead of the usual places, such as the hips or legs.[38] A study of women who were given estradiol after ovarian failure showed a reversal of this trend. This study demonstrated that supplemental estradiol reduced the percentage and amount of fat around the mid-section, thus reversing the imbalance in where fat is stored.[39] This imbalance cannot be restored by eating differently, or by exercise alone. Restoring ovarian hormonal balance would assist in reversing the abnormal balance of enzymes in the fat around the mid-section.

Worth noting also is that what makes the weight gain around the mid-section worse is that the muscles not only lose mass they lose tone. This means that the muscles are not as strong as they were during ovarian function and cannot keep the tummy as flat. The result is an even larger tummy.

Muscles contain receptors for estrogens, testosterone and progesterone, and these hormones are necessary for the muscles to work well. In fact 70 percent of the nuclei of muscle cells from the thigh muscles contain ER beta.[40] Remember that testosterone increases estrogen receptor beta expression. So, a decline in testosterone translates into a decline in estrogen receptor beta. Muscles can only work well if they get the "basic ingredients" that they require. And without ovarian hormones, they cannot get these "basic ingredients."

Muscles are important for several reasons. First, they provide us with the strength; and second, they increase metabolism by using more energy. Maintaining a good weight, with healthier fat distribution and stronger muscles, would reduce our risk for heart disease and diabetes and be a tremendous benefit of continued ovarian function.

SEXUAL RESPONSE

Ovarian hormones play a significant role in sexual response. Each woman knows what her own comfortable level of sexual response is. The level of each ovarian hormone required for comfortable sexual response however, varies depending on the individual. No matter what the level, a decline in ovarian function translates into a decline in sexual function. Preventing ovarian failure would avoid one cause of an imbalance in sex drive between lovers, which is created during and after ovarian failure. This imbalance can be disastrous for a sexual relationship. A woman can suffer a great deal of frustration and disappointment, as can her partner, when her body no longer responds to sexual stimuli.

Women who are living with ovarian failure are routinely counseled to just wait and be patient, and sexual response will return. Unfortunately, this simply is not true. To expect this to happen is also to expect the physiology of a woman's sex organs to change and begin to respond to sexual stimulation without adequate levels of sex hormones. This would mean that after ovarian failure the body would have to develop another mechanism to create the physical changes that occur during sexual activity. This way of thinking makes ovaries and their hormones superfluous to sexual response. Would this be said to a man that has sexual problems after castration? Just *wait* and your body will develop other mechanisms that will restore your ability to engage in sexual activity. Just *wait long enough* and once again you'll have normal erections and orgasms. No one would consider this a reasonable thing to say to a man, so what is reasonable about saying it to a woman?

Understanding the relationship between ovarian hormones and sexual response is important. We know what is necessary hormonally for sexual response to occur. In women, sex drive requires sufficient levels of two ovarian hormones to achieve sexual arousal and orgasm: estradiol and testosterone. Studies have been able to identify the minimum levels for most women to achieve sexual response. The minimum level of total estradiol is 50 pg/ml, and the minimum level of free testosterone is 2.0 pg/ml.[41, 42]

After ovarian failure the level of total estradiol falls, on average, to 12-20 pg/ml, and free testosterone falls to an average of 1.7 pg/ml. For some women free testosterone may be higher. However, without taking supplemental estradiol, levels of estradiol will never reach 50 pg/ml. This explains the distressing decrease in sexual response in women during and following ovarian failure.

Even with supplementation of estradiol, testosterone, or both to the minimum levels, sexual experience may still not be as satisfying as it was before ovarian failure. This may mean that either or both levels need to be higher. Yet even with higher levels, for some it may never be the same again. This is not because the body isn't capable of satisfactory sexual response; rather it is because we haven't figured out a way to balance the ovarian hormones as well as the ovaries can.

Generally, the level of total estradiol before ovarian failure is 50 to 200 pg/ml and free testosterone is 2.0 to 12.0 pg/ml, with a mid-range level of 6 pg/ml. Although it may take time to find the correct product and dose for each individual, sexual function can be substantially improved or restored if the decline in sexual response is due to low levels of estradiol and testosterone. Sometimes a topical testosterone cream and/or transdermal l-arginine product (such as Femoré™) applied directly to the clitoris and labia can be helpful in restoring sexual response. But replacing estradiol and testosterone still may not be everything that's needed. The ovaries produce many more hormones than just these. It could be that DHEA, which can break down into testosterone, may work better than testosterone itself. Very few studies have investigated the relationship between ovarian hormone replacement and female sexual response. Much more research is needed in this area.

One of the harshest parts of ovarian failure is realizing there is no difference between menopause and castration. By its very definition, there is no expectation of sexual response after castration. But if women are told that sexual function will return, does that mean that castration is different for women than it is for men? And if so, why don't doctors refer to women who've had their ovaries fail, as is the case in menopause, as castrated? Sexual activity is an important part of a marriage or sexual relationship. So when one partner literally loses the ability to participate in sexual activity this can put a strain on the relationship. For doctors to reassure women, and by extension their partners, that sexual response will return, without the benefit of normal levels of ovarian hormones, is wrong and unethical.

Clearly, being able to express one's feelings sexually over the course of a whole lifetime is a tremendous benefit to extending ovarian function into old age.

Women are told that ovarian failure is not a disease. This is true. Ovarian failure occurs because the ovaries have run out of eggs, nothing more. However, the loss of the ovaries *does* create and contribute to disease. Without question, women would be healthier with a lifetime of ovarian function than they would without it. It is time to be honest with ourselves, and it is time our doctors are honest with us, about the fallout of life without ovarian function. Ignoring the obvious doesn't make it go away.

HOT FLASHES AS AN EARLY INDICATOR OF OVARIAN FAILURE

Hot flashes are generally thought of as a benign reminder of failing ovaries. They're something you cannot ignore. Hot flashes are unmistakable and uncomfortable; they can be a persistent reminder of failing ovaries. Unfortunately, you cannot feel bone loss, or a hardening of the arteries or an increase in blood pressure, until the damage is done. A lack of hot flashes doesn't mean the ill effects of ovarian failure can be escaped. Hot flashes or not, these ill effects occur as a result of ovarian failure.

About 75 percent of women will get hot flashes as their ovaries begin to fail. Most women will suffer through them for about a year. For about 25 percent of women, however, these hot flashes continue for about 5 years. And some of us—about 5 percent—will experience them for decades, into old age. A hot flash generally begins in the upper body, usually around the chest, and then spreads to the arms, neck, and face. It can produce a large amount of perspiration and be very uncomfortable. Some women have as many as 60 hot flashes in a day. We do not know why they occur, but we do know that administering estradiol can help to relieve hot flashes in women and men.[43]

At the time of ovarian failure blood pressure begins to rise, which is a risk factor for heart disease. Hot flashes are a sign not only of failing ovaries, but also of the onset of increased blood pressure. Increased blood pressure is an established and important risk factor for heart disease. This increase in blood pressure can put a woman at a significantly increased risk of heart disease as her ovaries fail. Hot flashes may eventually resolve, but the increased blood pressure remains.

Key Points:
- Women outlive their ovaries
- Cancer risk goes up after ovarian failure
- Testosterone may protect against breast cancer
- Coronary artery disease is accelerated after ovarian failure
- The incidence of osteoporosis increases after ovarian failure
- Sleep becomes more difficult after ovarian failure
- Sexual function declines with ovarian failure
- Ovarian failure has a significant negative impact on a woman's body

CHAPTER 4

HOW TO PREVENT OVARIAN FAILURE

To prevent ovarian failure we need to understand exactly what it is. Ovarian failure is the term used to describe what happens when the ovaries exhaust their limited supply of eggs. As a woman ages and the supply of eggs in her ovaries goes down, the levels of ovarian hormones in her blood begin to change. As these changes occur, the rate at which the ovaries use their eggs increases, leading to the ovaries exhausting their supply of eggs sooner than they otherwise would have. By working to re-balance ovarian hormone levels, the rate at which the eggs are used can be corrected, allowing the supply of eggs to last 20 to 30 years longer.

A LIMITED SUPPLY OF EGGS

Unlike men who produce sperm throughout their adult life, women are born with all the eggs they will ever have. The eggs remain in the ovaries, unchanged, until they are called upon to mature and possibly be fertilized. Each month following the onset of menstruation, about 500 eggs will begin the approximately 6-month process of maturing. During the first two weeks of each menstrual cycle the batch of eggs recruited six months earlier reaches final maturation. However out of each month's batch of eggs, only one ovulates, traveling down the fallopian tube to the uterus for possible fertilization. The remaining eggs, which were recruited for a particular batch but did not ovulate, then die off (Figure 13). When a woman begins puberty it is estimated that the ovaries contain about half a million eggs each. It has further been

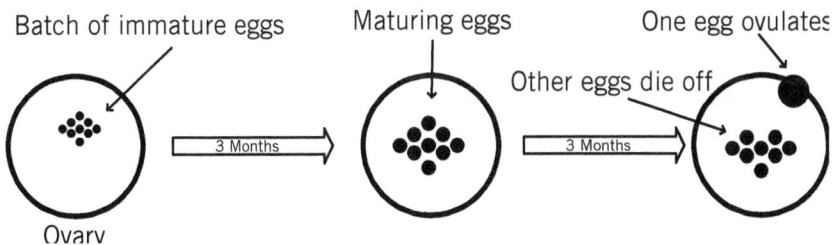

Figure 13: Egg maturation process takes many months

estimated that if these eggs were recruited at the same consistent rate, the supply would last a woman until her early 70's, which is about the same age that a man's testes begin to fail.

So what happens to all the other eggs? If there are enough to last for six decades, why do they only last for four? Under different circumstances could highly functioning ovaries last a lifetime, instead of just 40 years?

HOW OVARIES DEPLETE THEMSELVES TOO SOON

The monthly recruitment of eggs is done in a very tightly controlled hormonal feedback system, which involves the ovaries and two organs in the brain, the hypothalamus and the pituitary. In a feedback system if one level drops then another level rises to compensate. In this system the hormones produced by the ovary directly control the signals from the brain. If the ovary produces higher levels of hormones then the signal from the brain is lower.

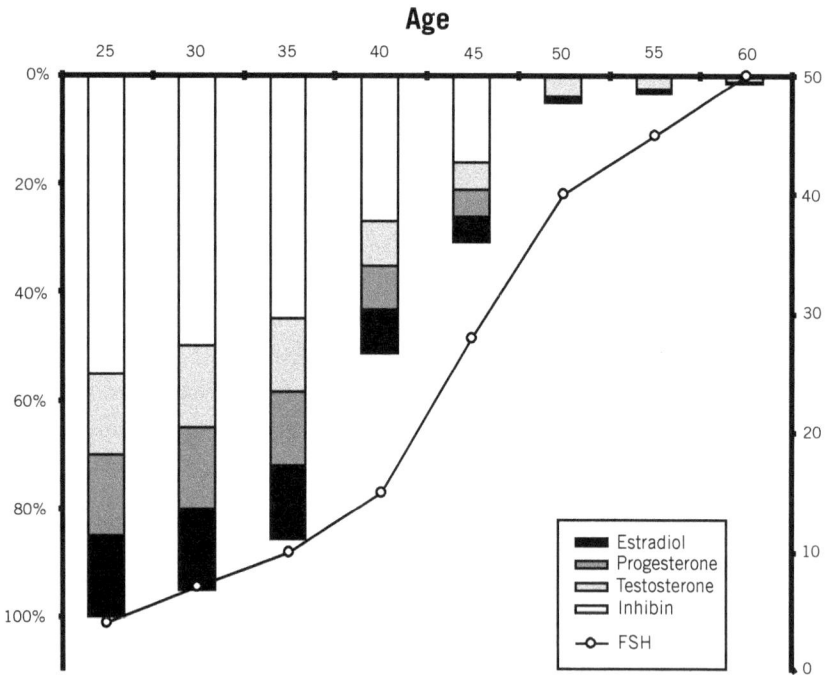

Figure 14: As levels of inhibin and testosterone fall, the level of FSH goes up; after ovarian failure, FSH continues to rise

Conversely, if the ovary produces lower levels of ovarian hormones then the signal from the brain rises. This "seesaw" between the ovary and the brain is what makes the menstrual cycle possible. The brain communicates with the ovary using a hormone called "follicle stimulating hormone," or FSH. And the ovaries, in turn, use estradiol, testosterone, progesterone and inhibin to communicate with the brain. Over time, the levels of two of the four ovarian hormones (testosterone and inhibin) drop.[1,2] And as a consequence, the level of FSH rises (see Figure 14). Estradiol levels drop dramatically close to the time that the ovaries completely fail. As the ovaries fail and less and less hormones are produced, the levels of FSH continue to rise. You can clearly see that without suppression, FSH continues to rise. This rise in FSH continues for the duration of a woman's life because there are no hormones being produced by the ovaries to stop it.

Estradiol and testosterone together suppress FSH levels only about 25 percent; progesterone about 15 percent; and inhibin about 60 percent.[3] Over time levels of testosterone and inhibin drop enough to allow FSH to rise substantially. As a result of this substantial rise in FSH a disruption occurs in how the eggs are recruited and matured[4]. With elevated levels of FSH, approximately twice as many eggs are recruited for each menstrual cycle. This accelerated use of eggs causes the ovaries to run out of eggs approximately 20 to 30 years sooner than they would with a steady recruitment of eggs.[5, 6, 7, 8] Given all the potential benefits of maintaining ovarian function, I think this is 20 to 30 years too soon.

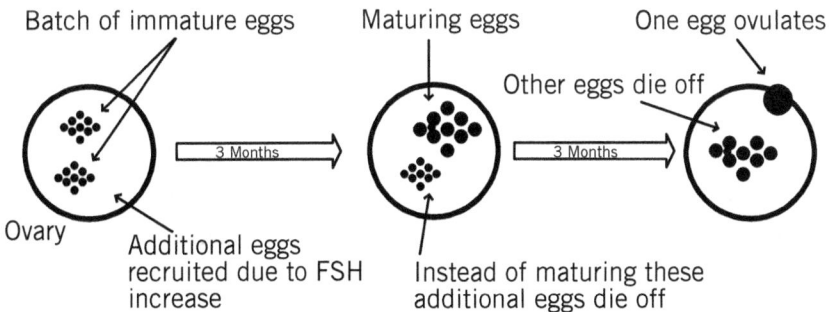

Figure 15: Egg recruitment with increased FSH

As FSH rises, there is an increase in the number of immature eggs, which enter the growing pool of eggs as shown in Figure 15. As levels of testosterone and inhibin are fairly constant, preventing a large rise in FSH by adding back very small amounts of testosterone and inhibin can be done easily. This would normalize ovarian function, and normal recruitment of eggs would be maintained. With normal recruitment of eggs the ovary would run out of eggs at about age 74 instead of age 50 (See Figure 16).[9, 10]

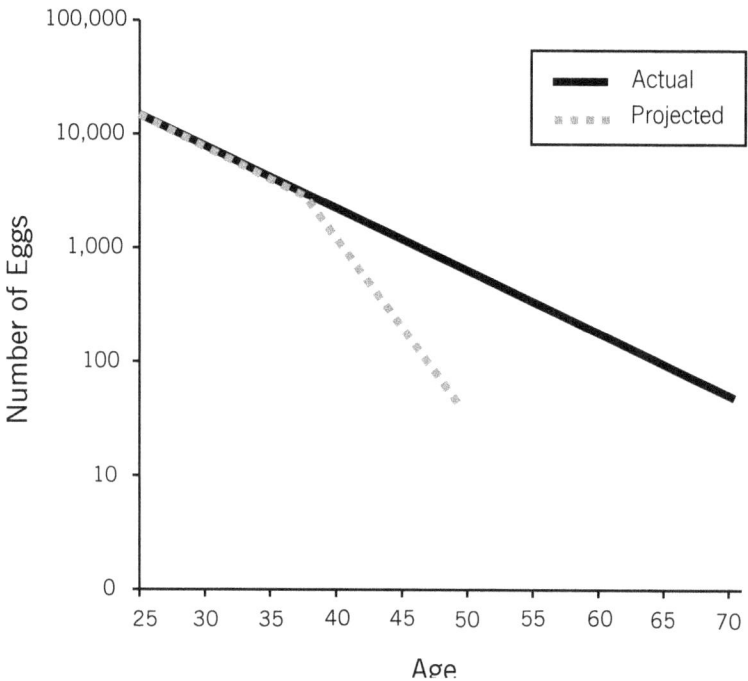

Figure 16: Eggs remaining in the ovaries by age

Understanding how eggs are recruited allows us to understand how ovaries are depleted decades too soon. Normalizing ovarian function, like normalizing the function of any other organ in the body, allows the organ to function for a longer period of time.

HOW THE LEVELS OF OVARIAN HORMONES CHANGE OVER TIME

As the level of FSH rises, the ovary is stimulated more than it normally would be, which results in higher than normal estradiol and progesterone levels.[11] Table 2 is a reference table of observed total and calculated free levels of estradiol, progesterone, testosterone and SHBG for women younger than age 30, between ages 30 to 40, 40 to 50, and after ovarian failure.[12, 13, 14, 15, 16, 17, 18] While the overall production of estradiol and progesterone increases as FSH rises, the level of testosterone falls. This is because the ovaries and the adrenal glands produce testosterone in about equal amounts. Between the ages of 25 and 30 the adrenal gland starts to produce less testosterone.[19] Combining levels of testosterone production from the ovaries with declining production from the adrenal glands results in an overall reduction in its level. This fall in production of testosterone by the adrenal glands contributes to the increase in FSH levels and premature depletion of the ovaries.

Age	Estradiol		Testosterone		Progesterone		SHBG
	Total (pg/ml)	Free (pg/ml)	Total (ng/dL)	Free (pg/ml)	Total (ng/ml)	Free (pg/ml)	(nM/L)
<30	30–300	3.3	40–100	6.0–15.0	11.0	330	40–60
30–40	40–300	3.4	30–80	4.5–12.0	12.4	372	50–70
40–50	50–300	3.5	25–50	3.0–7.5	13.8	414	60–80
>50 Ovarian Failure	12–20	.16	10–30	1.5–3.0	<0.5	15	80–110

Table 2: Reference table of observed hormone levels, free estradiol based on 2.0% and an average of 125-150 pg/ml for women with ovarian function and 1% free estradiol for women without ovarian function. Assume 1.5% free testosterone for women with ovarian function and about 1% for women without ovarian function. Assume 3.0% free progesterone.

RISK OF BIRTH DEFECTS

It has been shown that the risk of birth defects rises at the same time that levels of testosterone and inhibin begin to fall. We know that as FSH goes up a disruption in the recruitment and maturation of eggs occurs.[20] A result of this disruption is a decrease in fertility. The disruption worsens as FSH increases. In studies on women in their early 30's, a disruption in how eggs are matured can be seen along with a parallel increase in birth defects. The highest level of chromosomal birth defects occurs when FSH is at very high levels.[21] This can be seen in the risk of Down's syndrome, which increases concurrently with the rise of FSH (Figure 17). The question now is: Can birth defects be lowered by keeping FSH from rising, and normalizing ovarian function? And even with normalized ovarian function would the risk of birth defects be the same for an older woman? These are questions that only clinical studies can conclusively answer. At this point extending ovarian function may or may not increase birth defects. Would the risk of birth defects be dramatically lowered by using testosterone and inhibin to maintain appropriate levels of FSH? Until research is focused on this area, there are no clear answers.

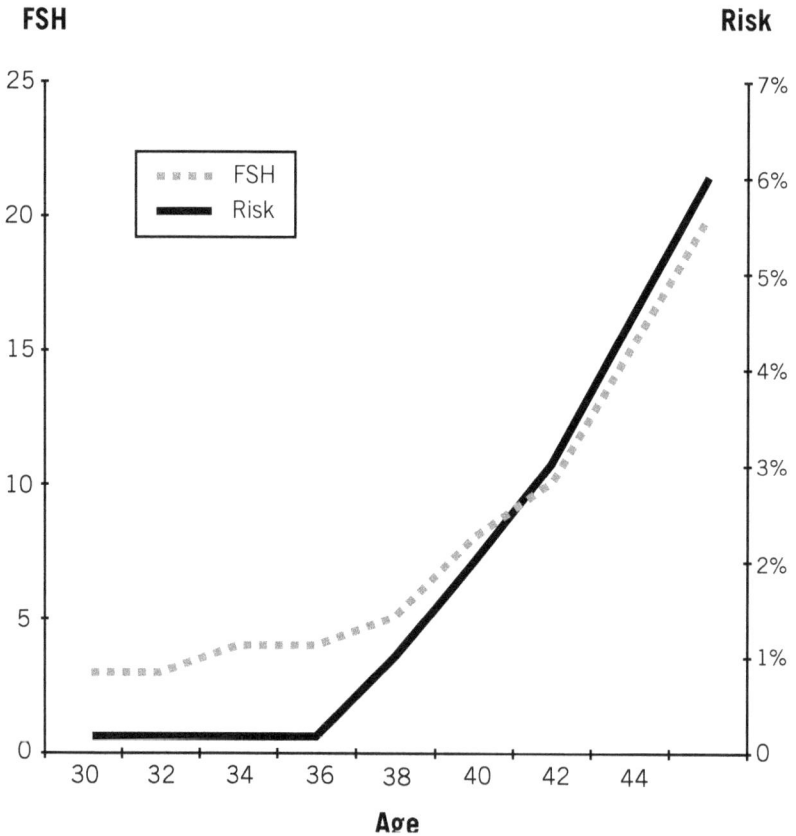

Figure 17: Risk of Down's syndrome and FSH vs. age

Testosterone helps the maturation of eggs in the earliest stages of their growth by stimulating the creation of FSH receptors (FSHr) directly on the eggs. As the eggs mature, these receptors help amplify the effect of FSH on the maturing eggs.[22, 23] A drop in androgen levels causes a decrease in the efficiency of this process.[24] The eggs within the ovaries are stored in a very primitive state. It is possible that over time the DNA within these eggs might change and become a source of birth defects. Currently, fertility drops sharply for women in their early 40's, but extending it by several decades may or may not increase birth defects. It would obviously be important to use the same screening methods for birth defects that we use now.

BIRTH CONTROL

With continued ovarian function a woman would need birth control that would be comfortable, and that would not cause birth defects if she were to get pregnant. Many contraceptives carry a risk of birth defects if a woman were to become pregnant. The reason this risk exists is that the oral contraceptive pill, the contraceptive patch, the contraceptive vaginal ring and progestin-only preparations contain hormones, which the growing fetus would not normally be exposed to in utero. Many of these hormones do not naturally occur within the body. For instance, instead of using an altered estrogen and an altered progesterone to suppress ovulation, inhibin and testosterone, which the body already produces naturally, could be used as an effective means of birth control. This combination was suggested as a form of birth control in the early 1980's. At that time it was proposed as an effective birth control method for men, as the combination is very effective in suppressing FSH and LH, which is necessary for creating temporary infertility.[25] Female and male birth control are based on the same premise however: suppressing FSH and LH. This form of birth control is thus a good idea for men *and* women.

Another advantage of using inhibin is that it does not alter the level of free testosterone, while effectively suppressing FSH. This is important, as the contraceptive pill, containing an oral estrogen, reduces the level of free testosterone by half. It does this by causing a large increase in the binding protein SHBG. Recall that testosterone may be very important in preventing breast cancer. Designing birth control with hormones that the body naturally produces, and that do not adversely affect other important hormone levels, will make birth control safer for women and for their unborn children.

PROTECTING YOUR OVARIES

If possible, any medication that can damage the eggs within the ovaries or change the hormonal balance, which can speed the depletion of eggs, should be avoided. Any medication that reduces estradiol or testosterone levels will remove some of the suppression of FSH, causing a disruption in the function of the ovaries and possibly lead to an early depletion of the ovaries. Any medication that reduces testosterone levels in men will reduce testosterone levels in women. And any medication that is toxic to the testes is toxic to the ovaries.

Surprisingly, oral contraceptive pills may help to deplete the ovaries prematurely. This is because the ovaries continue to recruit eggs even while on the pill. The pill does not allow any of these eggs to mature fully and ovulate, thus protecting a woman from becoming pregnant. Oral contraceptives do suppress FSH; however, all oral contraceptives reduce free testosterone levels by at least half. Reducing the free testosterone level upsets the delicate hormonal balance that controls how many eggs are recruited per menstrual cycle. More eggs are recruited per cycle, and thus the net results is an earlier onset of ovarian failure. An observational study done in the Netherlands found that for every year of oral contraceptive use, ovarian failure would occur 1.2 months sooner.[26] This implies that if a woman has been on the pill for 20 years she can expect an earlier onset of ovarian failure by about 2 years.

Women with higher testosterone levels tend to have a later onset of ovarian failure. This makes sense, as higher testosterone levels mean that FSH is suppressed for a longer period of time. This allows the normal recruitment of eggs to be maintained longer as women continue to age. Women who are slightly overweight tend to have measurably higher free testosterone levels than normal weight or underweight women, as do women who exercise. Women who are overweight have a slightly different balance of enzymes, which result in higher levels of free testosterone. One of the reasons women who exercise have higher free testosterone levels is that during the period of time that they are exercising, and shortly after, blood flow is diverted from their liver to their muscles. Hormones are broken down in the liver, so less blood flow to the liver means less testosterone is broken down—and more stays in the bloodstream.[27]

Many substances, such as cigarette smoke, chemotherapy drugs, and alcohol, are toxic to the ovaries. Long-term exposure to these substances will damage the ovaries and cause an early onset of ovarian failure. It has been documented that smoking in particular causes an earlier onset of ovarian failure by one to two years.[28] Smoking causes the binding protein of testosterone (sex-hormone binding globulin, or SHBG) to increase.[29, 30] Recall that an increase in SHBG means a decrease in free testosterone. Many medications also raise SHBG levels.[31] Maintaining a tightly controlled feedback loop between the ovaries and the brain is the best way to maintain normal ovarian function throughout your life.

The medical community is beginning to understand that ovaries can be protected from the harmful effects of chemotherapy, which is used to treat many different kinds of cancer. This is being shown in important clinical trials that are currently in progress, trials that were designed solely to reduce the amount of damage done to ovaries during chemotherapy. Instead of administering chemotherapy and hoping that the ovaries aren't too heavily damaged, a medication is given which reduces FSH to very low levels, which suppresses the functioning of the ovaries. *Then* chemotherapy is given. Ovarian suppression is continued for a period of time after chemotherapy stops. One of these trials is already showing less damage to the ovaries during chemotherapy than what would normally be observed, had nothing been done. So far the results of this trial have been very good. All the women using ovarian suppression medication retained ovarian function after chemotherapy; while all the women not using it suffered severe ovarian damage.[32] In another trial women had similarly good results.[33] These trials highlight the fact that preserving ovarian function is possible.[34, 35] However, depending on the type of cancer being treated, patients will still need to have a serious discussion with their doctors about the risks and benefits associated with maintaining long-term ovarian function.

Earlier ovarian failure has also been documented in women alcoholics. This is because chronic alcoholism can damage the liver. Liver damage can negatively influence the delicate hormonal balance that controls how the ovaries work. Chronic alcoholism causes similar irreversible damage to the testes.[36, 37]

Now you can see that ovarian failure, or menopause, may potentially be prevented. The idea is not only to have ovarian function and the resultant health benefits for a lifetime, but also to potentially reduce the incidence of birth defects and perhaps extend the number of years that a woman can have a healthy baby. Women should be offered treatment to help their ovaries work at an optimal level for as long as possible. Women should be given a choice to live their lives with or without ovarian function.

Key Points:

- Women have a limited supply of eggs
- Ovaries deplete themselves at an accelerated rate as a woman ages
- Ovarian hormone levels change as a woman ages
- Risk of birth defects goes up as levels of FSH rise
- You need to protect your ovaries so that they function for as many years as possible

CHAPTER 5

RESTORING THE BALANCE

Extending the functional life of the ovary means restoring the balance of ovarian hormones that work to control it. This means identifying what the "right" right balance is. The balance you try to achieve will be based on your personal goals. Whatever goals and balance you choose, you need to use the right hormones, delivered the right way, for your situation. Only then will you be in a position to successfully take advantage of the health benefits of proper ovarian hormonal balance.

HOW TO RESTORE NORMAL OVARIAN HORMONAL BALANCE

The goal at any age is to regulate ovarian function, and if that is not possible, then to restore normal ovarian hormonal balance. At about age 30 ovarian function begins to change.[1] This disruption in function is called ovarian dysregulation. With it comes an increase in the rate of birth defects and an increase in the risk for breast cancer and heart disease, as well as other ill effects on the body.

Communication between the brain and the ovaries is best when their "seesaw," the way they interact and affect one another (see page 54), is working well. This "seesaw" works best when appropriate levels of estradiol, testosterone, progesterone and inhibin are all available and working together to suppress levels of FSH. Without suppression, FSH levels continue to rise. As long as the ovary continues to function normally, estradiol and progesterone levels remain steady. Over time there is a drop in overall testosterone levels because of the reduced output of testosterone from the adrenal glands. Over time there is also a drop in inhibin from the ovary. To normalize function, and keep recruitment of eggs steady, it would be necessary to replace both testosterone and inhibin. Unfortunately, it is only possible to replace testosterone, as inhibin is not currently available to women. Replacing testosterone to youthful levels may add some longevity to ovarian function. This is because suppression of FSH longer would allow the ovary to work for a longer period of time (see page 68). If the ovaries have already failed, and are non-responsive, then a balance of youthful levels of ovarian hormones to maintain the health benefits of functioning ovaries can be used.

It is important to keep in mind that all the ovarian hormones may not have to be added back; however, be prepared that this may be necessary. Transitioning from the use of hormones produced by the ovaries to supplemental hormones should be overseen by someone who is very familiar with the different types of products available. He or she should also know how to administer them in a way that is most convenient for the woman in question, and most compatible with how her body works. Assisting women in maintaining ovarian hormone balance throughout their adult lives is the type of work appropriate to an Ovarian Specialist (see page 77).

DEFINE YOUR GOALS

Different hormones are used to normalize ovarian function and restore ovarian hormones after ovarian failure. If the ovaries haven't yet failed, use testosterone and inhibin (as shown in Table 3) to maintain appropriate levels. Once the ovaries are normalized, you can also expect normal levels of estradiol and progesterone. Once the ovaries have failed, use Table 4 to determine the levels of hormones that must be maintained to achieve your various goals.

Whether a woman has a uterus or not, progesterone is a necessary part of restoring ovarian hormonal balance to the body.[2] This is because progesterone receptors are located throughout the body, not just in the uterus. Progesterone has also been shown to be as effective as estradiol in relaxing blood vessels, which can help to prevent heart disease. On page 79 ("Understanding Your Laboratory Report") I include suggested minimum levels of testosterone and estradiol to prevent "estradiol starvation" of the breast tissue. As discussed in this section, it is important to use an accurate laboratory test (such as an equilibrium dialysis or equilibrium ultrafiltration) when monitoring these levels.[3, 4]

For:	Free Estradiol	Free Testosterone	Free Progesterone	Inhibin	FSH
Maintaining Ovarian Function (suggested)	2 pg/ml day 5	6.0 pg/ml day 3–5	275 pg/ml day 21	240 pg/l day 3–5	<6.0 day 3–5

Table 3: Recommended hormone levels prior to ovarian failure

For:	Free Estradiol	Free Testosterone	Free Progesterone
Prevention of Osteoporosis	0.20 pg/ml	6.0 pg/ml	
Sexual Function	1–4 pg/ml	2.0–12.0 pg/ml (mid-range 6 pg/ml)	
Restoring Ovarian Hormonal Balance (suggested)	2 pg/ml	6.0 pg/ml	275 pg/ml day 21

Table 4: Recommended hormone levels after ovarian failure

OVARIAN HORMONE PRODUCTS

Your goal will help you decide which combination of products is best for you. See Table 5 for a list of the pros and cons of oral and transdermal preparations.[5] Only the effects on levels of free rather than total estradiol and testosterone are listed. It is generally accepted that only the free portion of any hormone is active in the body, while the bound portion is inactive.

Remember that estradiol taken orally will increase the binding protein (SHBG), which holds estradiol and testosterone in the bloodstream. In some women it may also increase HDL, the good cholesterol. However do keep in mind that taking any estrogen orally may also increase levels of triglycerides, which is a risk factor for heart disease and diabetes. This increase in triglycerides may lead to a decrease in HDL (instead of the expected increase of HDL).

	Free Estradiol	Free Testosterone	Triglycerides	HDL	
Estradiol, Oral	↑	↓half the level	↑or ↓	↑or↓	May Increase Risk of Diabetes
Estradiol, Transdermal	↑	same	same	same	
Testosterone, Oral	↑	↑		↓	Increased Risk of Liver Cancer
Testosterone, Transdermal	same	↑		↓	

Table 5: Effects of delivery method on hormone level

A further consideration is that an increase in SHBG will decrease the free amount of estradiol and testosterone. So unless you want to reduce the amount of free estradiol and free testosterone, it is best to use a transdermal estradiol cream or patch.

There are very few choices for dosage with a patch, and thus it may be necessary to use multiple patches to reach your goal. For example, the .1 mg estradiol patch may raise your level of estradiol anywhere from 17 to 195 pg/ml. This is a very wide range and is not influenced by weight.[6] It only takes about a day to reach a steady level, so a blood test two days after applying a patch will tell you how well the estradiol is being absorbed through your skin.

There is also an estradiol cream approved by the FDA, and soon there will be an estradiol gel. The cream has a large variability in absorption. Dosages for a patch are not the same as dosages for a cream. For instance, wearing a .1 mg patch is not the same as applying .1 mg estradiol from a cream. This is because the patch delivers estradiol very slowly over a period of a day. The patch is closely adhered to the skin. Very little of the estradiol is lost and most is absorbed. Spreading a cream over an area of skin allows a great deal of loss of estradiol, so much larger amounts must be used to absorb the same amount of estradiol as you would with a patch.

As a general rule, expect about 3.5 g of estradiol cream (Estrasorb™) to raise your level of estradiol to about 50 pg/ml.[7] If you are using a compounded cream made by a pharmacist, request a vanishing cream base, as it absorbs slower and will create a steady level of estradiol over a longer period of time. Estradiol has a short half-life. Thus it is likely it will need to be applied twice a day to maintain steady levels of estradiol.

A patch is also important for the delivery of progesterone, because when progesterone is delivered in pill or cream form it can be absorbed too quickly and cause extreme drowsiness. At night this side effect might prove beneficial but during the day, obviously, it can pose problems. With current technology, a progesterone patch would need to be a little bigger than the smallest estradiol patch, and would have to be changed daily for 14 days each month.[8] However with improved technology, an extended wear patch could certainly be a reality. This is important to remember—a progesterone patch *can* be developed. Whether or not it will ever be made available depends largely on the pharmaceutical industry's interest in recognizing and meeting this need.

Unfortunately, there are currently no approved testosterone or inhibin products for women. Testosterone can be made by a compounding pharmacy, and testosterone products made for men may be useful for women. A compounding pharmacy will make custom creams and pills as per a doctor's prescription. There may soon be another option: a testosterone patch made for women. Currently the testosterone patch is only being marketed to improve sexual function. It is formulated to last three to four days and works by releasing very small amounts of testosterone over that time period. The resultant levels of testosterone are within the normal pre-menopausal range.

Testosterone is also available in pills, creams, lozenges (troches) or gels. In studies on testosterone replacement for women, closest to normal testosterone levels seem to be best achieved by a patch or gel. The optimal choice is one that is both convenient and effective. As a general rule 1 mg of testosterone in a cream or gel will raise your testosterone level by approximately 25 ng/dl. However no matter what method you choose to achieve a satisfying level of free testosterone, it may be that the total testosterone is higher than the recommended range (<86 ng/dl). Focus on the free testosterone range first to obtain your goals. And, try to keep the total testosterone under 100 ng/dl, if possible. Until products designed specifically for women are made available, the use of men's products may result in higher total and free testosterone levels than are normally seen in women.

Increased hair on the body (hirsutism) and other male characteristics are always a concern when using testosterone products. Remember that you're only replacing what your ovaries once made, and that your body recognizes testosterone and will use it appropriately. Your body was designed to use testosterone and needs it to function well. It may be that you get a few pimples or acne, but do understand that the dose can be adjusted. Just remember that if you never got many pimples in the past and you feel normal on the dose that you're getting in the present, then it is very unlikely that you'll begin to grow a beard or develop a deeper voice. It is actually far more likely that a lack of ovarian hormone balance will produce masculine traits. Without the influence of normal levels of estradiol, even a little bit of testosterone over time can cause a deepening of the voice and an increase in hair production, particularly on the face.

Currently there is only one FDA approved progesterone product available: Prometrium™, and it is taken orally. Many products are called progesterones; however only this one is actually identical to human progesterone. The others are made from testosterone or progesterone molecules, which are chemically manipulated to function enough like progesterone to cause a period (menstrual flow). Prometrium™ is an important product, as it is the only bio-identical progesterone available. While it represents an important breakthrough—as will the testosterone patch—it does have its drawbacks. For instance, it can be very sedating. Prometrium™ can cause progesterone levels to be very high—about two to five times higher, depending on the dosage, than normal progesterone levels. Taking Prometrium™ with food increases its absorption, and results in blood levels double those achieved when taking it on an empty stomach. This can intensify any side effects, such as extreme drowsiness.[9] The drawbacks of Prometrium™ highlight the lack of appropriate products available for restoring normal ovarian hormonal balance. However, even with these drawbacks, Prometrium™ is bio-identical to human progesterone and is far superior to any patented progestin.

It takes time for the body to adapt to any change in dosage, so allow yourself a two to four week adjustment period. And rest assured that a balance *can* be found.

NORMALIZING OVARIAN FUNCTION

A balance of ovarian hormones is necessary to ensure the slow and steady release of eggs from the ovaries. As long as the release of eggs is slow and steady, a woman should have enough eggs to last her into her 70's, at least. It is a good idea to begin to have ovarian hormone levels checked as early as age 30. I believe that supplementing the levels of inhibin and/or testosterone would maintain optimum levels (see Table 3). If the ovaries are functioning normally, then normal levels of estradiol and progesterone will be produced and therefore will not need to be replaced. It is only the testosterone produced by the adrenal glands and the inhibin that is produced by the ovaries that I believe needs to be replaced (see Figure 18). Studies should be done to confirm that the supplementation of these two hormones can postpone menopause by decades—essentially preventing menopause during a woman's lifetime.

Probably the best way to increase the testosterone level is by using a testosterone patch, as it introduces steady levels of testosterone throughout the day without any highs or lows. Other ways to supplement testosterone levels would include using a testosterone gel or cream or even oral DHEA, as it is better absorbed orally than through the skin. As you know, at this time there are no commercially available testosterone preparations for women (see page

66). It is important to keep testosterone and inhibin as close to normal to keep FSH at appropriate levels (see Figure 19). Fortunately, there is now a way to see that efforts in restoring ovarian function are successful, since the volume of the ovaries can be measured using an ultrasound. Based on the volume, a doctor can calculate the time when the ovaries will be depleted, and will fail.[10] So, you now have the tools to ensure that you have ovarian function over the course of your entire lifetime.

Too much testosterone could be harmful to a fetus should a woman get pregnant while using supplemental testosterone. A testosterone patch made for women is currently undergoing clinical trials and, if approved, will unfortunately only be available in two doses. It may be that a woman needs a different dose than will be available to restore a slow and steady retrieval of eggs. If the dose needed is not readily available, a compounded cream made by a pharmacist can be used. Inhibin is also currently unavailable to the public. However, it is routinely used for research purposes. Ironically, the purpose

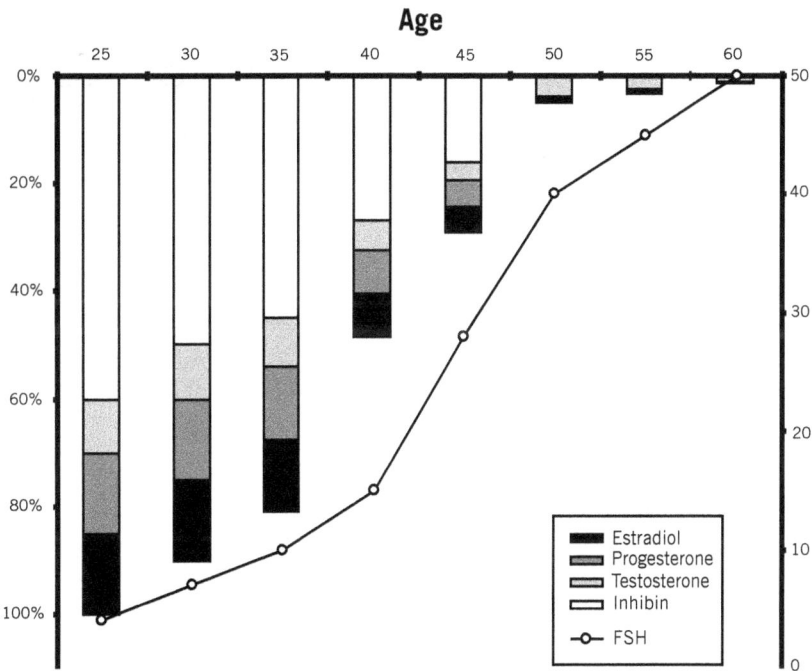

Figure 18: Unsupplemented ovarian function

of this research is to learn more about reproduction in men, and not women. A call for its availability was made over 20 years ago by researchers who wanted to create birth control for men using a combination of inhibin and testosterone.[11] Ultimately it is up to the pharmaceutical industry to recognize the importance of normalizing ovarian function, and to produce the necessary products for women to use.

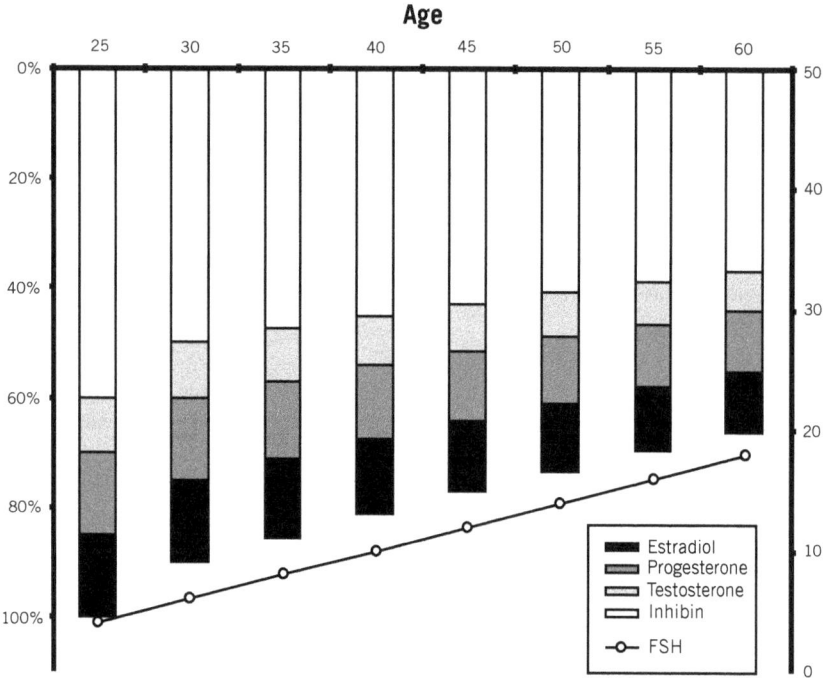

Figure 19: Normalized ovarian function with supplemental inhibin and testosterone

Key Points:
- It is important to restore ovarian hormonal balance for optimal health benefits
- You need to know your goal before you begin restoring ovarian hormone levels
- Choose the right products for your situation
- Normalizing ovarian function is key to the longevity of the ovaries

UNDERSTANDING STANDARD HORMONE REPLACEMENT THERAPY AS USED IN THE WOMEN'S HEALTH INITIATIVE

Standard hormone replacement therapy is an oral estrogen (typically Premarin™) and a progestin (typically Provera™). The term hormone replacement therapy (HRT) is deceptive. It suggests that the hormones produced by the ovaries are being replaced. We know that the ovaries produce estradiol, testosterone and progesterone. Since standard HRT contains an oral estrogen and a progestin, one would assume that at least estradiol and progesterone are being replaced. In fact, standard HRT contains only minimal amounts of estradiol, and cuts free testosterone levels by at least half, creating a hormonal balance that is lower than is found after ovarian failure. Standard HRT, of the sort used for the last 75 years, was never intended to replace ovarian hormones. After taking standard HRT estradiol is still in the ovarian failure range, as are testosterone and progesterone.

The Women's Health Initiative (WHI) was a large clinical trial designed in the early 1990's to test the effectiveness of a particular regimen. Standard HRT was used in the WHI for the purpose of increasing HDL, a good cholesterol, and decreasing bone loss. Until I wrote this book I, like most women, thought that hormone replacement therapy would replace ovarian hormones. I had always tucked away in the back of my mind the notion that I would use hormone replacement therapy when my ovaries failed. And I expected that this set of hormones would enable me to continue living the life I had prior to ovarian failure. I had no reason to think otherwise. I had no reason to expect that the Women's Health Initiative would fail. Rather, I had every reason to look forward to it succeeding—reducing the risk of heart disease and cancer, and maintaining quality of life.

WHAT I FOUND

I was quite surprised, therefore, when one arm of the Women's Health Initiative was cancelled in July 2002. It made no sense to me that the same hormones that were responsible for protecting a woman's body *before* ovarian failure could be what failed to protect a woman afterwards, making her more vulnerable to disease. I dismissed the failure of the WHI as politics and decided to continue believing that standard hormone replacement was right for me, and that when my ovaries failed me I would use standard HRT as planned.

But news reports continued to trickle in, making it more and more apparent that standard hormone replacement therapy was unhealthy for women. Not only was standard hormone replacement not going to prevent heart disease, it slightly increased the risk of breast cancer. With so many negative reports I could no longer dismiss the ill effects of HRT as just politics.

This made no sense. How could the same body that functioned so well *with* ovarian hormones change the way it functioned—and reject the very hormones that protected it from disease? I began reading about the regimens of hormones that were given to women so that I could see for myself what was going on. I read editorials in the *New England Journal of Medicine* and the *Journal of the American Medical Association*, and I studied the "Design of the Women's Health Initiative Clinical Trial and Observational Study." But I still could not see a clear reason for the trial's results. If ovarian hormones were replaced, why did a woman's health decline?

I decided to take a closer look at the regime of hormones given in the WHI. I had always assumed that "hormone replacement therapy" meant replacing the specific ovarian hormones, and so I compared the levels of ovarian hormones for functioning ovaries, ovarian failure, and with WHI HRT. It surprised me to see that what was given was less a hormone replacement therapy and more a liver medication. As I reviewed the purpose of the Women's Health Initiative the reasons for this started making more sense.

THE GOALS OF THE WHI

In the document entitled "Design of the Women's Health Initiative Clinical Trial and Observational Study," the following statement explains the purpose of this clinical trial:

> "The Women's Health Initiative (WHI) is a large and complex clinical investigation of strategies for the prevention and control of some of the most common causes of morbidity and mortality among postmenopausal women, including cancer, cardiovascular disease, and osteoporotic fractures."

In the same document the following explanation was given for the dosage chosen:

> "The dose of 0.625 mg/day was chosen because it is considered the minimum effective dose for the preservation of bone mineral density. This dose has been demonstrated to lead to a significant rise in HDL cholesterol and drop in LDL cholesterol."[1]

The designers of this clinical trial wanted to prevent and control heart disease, colon cancer and osteoporosis and tried to do so by using only one medication. They needed a medication that would cause the liver to produce more HDL and offer enough estradiol to offer protection from osteoporosis. An oral estrogen can do both. A minimal dose of oral estrogen can marginally increase estradiol levels and still be in the ovarian failure range, and at the same time cause the liver to increase production of HDL.[2, 3]

WHAT THE WHI ACTUALLY DID

To appreciate how different the hormone replacement therapy used in the original design of the Women's Health Initiative is from ovarian function, take a look at the following graphs (Figure 20 and Figure 21). They represent total and free estradiol, testosterone and progesterone levels.[2, 3, 4, 5] These graphs compare the highest levels reached during menopause; treatment with Premarin™ only; and normal pre-menopausal levels. Looking at these levels of ovarian hormones illustrates that the goal of this trial was not to raise estradiol, testosterone or progesterone to ovarian function levels, but to prevent

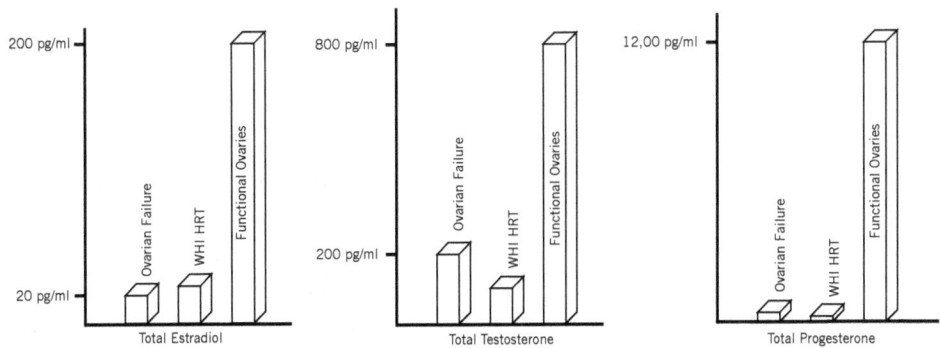

Figure 20: Total ovarian hormone comparison

heart disease by manipulating the liver into producing more HDL by using an oral estrogen to stimulate its production and halt bone loss. The resultant levels of estradiol are virtually the same as found in ovarian failure, and the resultant levels of testosterone and progesterone are lower than those found in ovarian failure. Calling this set of hormones hormone replacement therapy makes it sound like the hormones of the ovaries are being replaced.

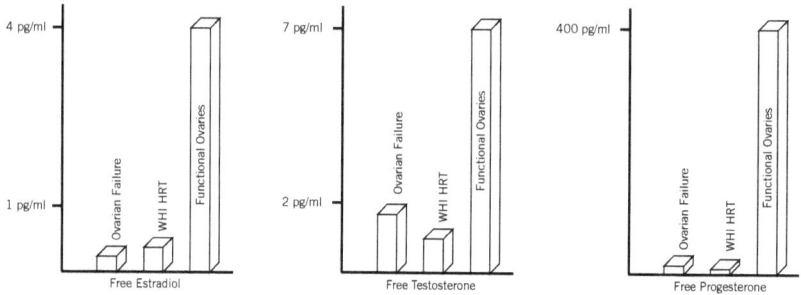

Figure 21: Free ovarian hormone comparison

After HRT the resultant level of estradiol for women is still what it would be for men. It is only for those called "high responders" that estradiol levels reach the lowest end of the levels of estradiol for men (see Figure 22: Estradiol levels).

Remember that the range of estradiol for a man is 25 to 50 pg/ml. After ovarian failure the range of estradiol for a woman is 12 to 20 pg/ml. After HRT the level is only about 15 to 28 pg/ml. The lowest point of the menstrual cycle for estradiol is 30 pg/ml. The range for prepubescent is 8 to 12 pg/ml.

Later in the trial all women either received an estrogen and a progestin if they had a uterus, only an estrogen if they did not, or a placebo. The estrogen pill was Premarin™ and the progestin was Medroxyprogesterone™. As is the case with any medications, Premarin™ and Medroxyprogesterone™ have side effects. Like any oral estrogen the expected side effects include breast tenderness, weight gain, headache, and irregular bleeding, as well as an increase in triglycerides and C-Reactive Protein, or CRP (both of which are risk factors for heart disease), and an increase in the binding protein for all of the ovarian and thyroid hormones.[6, 7, 8] The increase in binding protein means a decrease in the free level of these hormones. All of these side effects

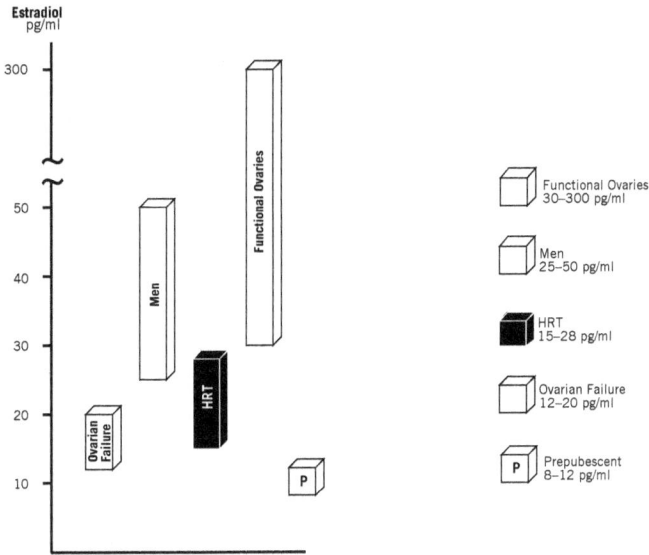

Figure 22: Estradiol levels

contribute to why the majority of women, across all socio-economic strata, discontinue use of HRT within 6 to 12 months.[9]

Unfortunately a decrease in free testosterone may also mean an increase in the risk of breast cancer via an increase in ER alpha (see page 39: "How Testosterone May Protect Against Breast Cancer"). This may further increase the risk of breast cancer beyond what is normally seen in ovarian failure. The decrease in testosterone also leads to a decrease in bone density.

All estrogens are known to increase the risk of uterine cancer. To reduce this risk Medroxyprogesterone™ was given on a monthly cycle, which resulted in a monthly bleed. This protected the uterus from any build-up that may have occurred as a result of taking Premarin™. Unfortunately, Medroxyprogesterone™ decreases HDL by about 15 to 20 percent, which completely negates the positive effect of the Premarin™ on HDL. It also significantly decreases testosterone levels—and this is in addition to the decrease caused by the Premarin™.[10, 11, 12, 13] Unfortunately Medroxyprogesterone™ has also been shown to negate the positive effect estrogen has on vasodilation, which increases the risk of vasospasm, thus increasing the risk of heart attack.[14, 15] The FDA has allowed the combination of Premarin™ and Medroxyprogesterone™ to be called hormone *replacement* therapy, which implies that this

75

combination is based on replacement of the ovarian hormones. In fact, it contains only minimal amounts of the hormones made by functional ovaries. Premarin™ contains a very small amount of estradiol, and a token amount of a precursor hormone that must be converted to estradiol once it is digested.[16] Premarin™ also decreases the levels of free progesterone that are produced by the adrenal gland—to levels lower than those found in ovarian function and ovarian failure. Together, Premarin™ and Medroxyprogesterone™ lower testosterone to levels not normally seen either during ovarian function or after ovarian failure. Medroxyprogesterone™ is a chemically altered progesterone molecule which can cause a period, but does not function like progesterone in other parts of the body.[12]

In short, Premarin™ and Medroxyprogesterone™ create an artificial hormonal balance, which does not normally occur during a woman's lifetime, either before or after ovarian failure. It is important to understand that the goal of this combination of medications was to prevent heart disease by improving the lipid profile and decreasing bone loss. It was never intended to replace ovarian hormonal balance. This makes it completely misleading to refer to it as hormone replacement therapy. We already know that women suffer ill health when they suffer ovarian failure. To make those levels even lower and expect better health is counterintuitive and illogical. Knowing this, it is easier to understand the results of the Women's Health Initiative—particularly once you understand that it was not based at all on ovarian hormone balance, but rather on elements of lipid (fat) and bone metabolism.

Key Points:
- The Woman's Health Initiative did not restore ovarian hormonal levels
- The goal of the WHI was to prevent heart disease, cancer and osteoporosis, and not to replace any ovarian hormones
- The hormones given in the WHI had adverse affects on other natural hormone levels
- The hormone levels created by the WHI do not occur naturally either before or after ovarian failure

CHAPTER 7

WORKING WITH YOUR MEDICAL PROFESSIONAL

To prevent ovarian failure and to be able to recreate the hormonal balance produced by the ovaries would require a different focus in current medical practice. It is thus important that both you and your doctor agree on the same goals. You will not only need to know how to read the results of your laboratory tests, but also understand the limitations of those tests. Again, it is absolutely crucial that you and your doctor agree on your course of treatment. It is not enough to say you want to normalize your ovarian function or recreate ovarian hormone balance. Your doctor may have another interpretation of normalizing or recreating ovarian balance. Remember that unless you are very clear, it is very likely you will be given standard HRT (Premarin™ and Medroxyprogesterone™). Standard HRT does not replace ovarian hormones, but rather creates ovarian hormone levels that are even lower than those seen in ovarian failure. Standard HRT was never intended to replace ovarian hormones.

You must be very clear about what it is you want. You need to know what levels you are trying to attain, and follow up with blood tests to verify that you have reached your goals. It is unfortunate that you cannot simply say: *I want to replace my ovarian hormones.* It is your responsibility to make sure you reach your goals. Since inhibin is unavailable at this time, you can only use testosterone to replace falling levels to help suppress FSH. If your doctor is unwilling to work with you, explain that testosterone, like estradiol, has been shown to suppress FSH. Explain that your goal is to extend the functional life of your ovaries, and that you need help to do that. If your doctor continues to be unwilling to work with you then you will have to find a new doctor.

OVARIAN SPECIALISTS

The focus of this new type of practice would be to treat ailments of the ovary, as well as to prevent ovarian failure by preventing the premature depletion of eggs and maintaining ovarian hormonal balance for women throughout their lives. To fill this need in women's healthcare I propose that a new specialty—the practitioners of which would be called Ovarian Specialists or OS for short—be created.

This would be a specialty that requires the knowledge of an endocrinologist and a gynecologist, with the additional knowledge of how the ovarian hormones interact with every major organ system in the body, as well as an understanding of how medications can affect the functioning of the ovaries. An OS would focus on tracking the declining function of a woman's ovaries and restoring her optimal ovarian hormonal balance in order to maintain optimal levels of overall function and egg usage as she ages.

An OS would work with pharmaceutical firms to improve drug delivery methods of ovarian hormones. The OS would also identify medications that disrupt the balance of ovarian hormones in the body, and cause harm to the long-term health of the ovaries. An OS would work with pharmaceutical firms to create the first ever progesterone patch. The progesterone patch would be able to create progesterone levels that are more similar to the levels produced naturally by the ovaries—more similar than the levels produced with a progesterone pill or any currently available cream. This would give the OS more tools with which to maintain or restore a proper balance of ovarian hormones.

An OS would understand how all the organs in the body are affected on a cellular level by both ovarian function and the loss of ovarian function. The OS would understand that a "one size fits all" approach does not work when it comes to restoring ovarian hormonal balance. The OS would work with each patient to develop an individualized treatment plan that works best for that patient.

An OS would combine the necessary knowledge of ovarian function (as it pertains to the specialties of gynecology, internal medicine, gastroenterology, oncology, orthopedics, pulmonology and endocrinology) with an appreciation for the role that ovarian health plays in preventing breast cancer, heart disease and bone loss, and maintaining sexual health. An ovarian specialist would know how to address problems that arise in the body that are directly related to failing or failed ovaries, and how to treat these problems. He or she would be able to fill that critical gap in medical practice, where, currently, ovarian health is not even a real consideration. You can help make the subspecialty of Ovarian Specialist a reality.

UNDERSTANDING YOUR LABORATORY REPORT

To monitor your own levels of ovarian hormones, you will need to understand your laboratory reports. Normal levels of hormones are always listed on laboratory reports, along with the results. Unfortunately, the medical community has not established standard levels for what is normal. Each laboratory determines its own normal levels, which are merely the statistical average of the results of the tests that it runs. This means that each laboratory determines its own reference range. To further complicate matters, many laboratories still continue to use older, unreliable methods of testing, and have not updated their methods to more modern and reliable techniques.[1, 2, 3]

Laboratories offer tests for total and free levels of many hormones. At this time, however, doctors routinely only request tests for free testosterone, not free estradiol or free progesterone. Even the testosterone tests have their problems when it comes to measuring women's hormone levels. Because the most commonly used test for measuring free testosterone was originally developed for men (who have much higher free and total testosterone levels than women), its accuracy for women is not reliable. This is a situation that must be rectified if we are to adequately address the problem of ovarian failure.[4]

The three tests used to measure free testosterone are: RIA, equilibrium ultrafiltration and equilibrium dialysis. The RIA method, which is most commonly used, is less accurate and more inconsistent than either of the other methods. There is also no way to compare RIA results to the results of other methods due to the inconsistencies of RIA—though as a general rule levels determined by the RIA method are two to three times lower than the more accurate methods. The normal range listed for the RIA method is approximately 0.0 to 3.9 pg/ml, and for the other methods it is approximately 1.0 to 8.5 pg/ml (see Table 6).[5, 6, 7] Most laboratories will perform the RIA test unless another method is specifically requested. All levels of free testosterone referenced in this book are based on the more accurate ultrafiltration or dialysis methods, as both of these are consistent and comparable. They are also the preferred tests used for scientific research. Most papers written about women's testosterone levels report levels obtained using either the ultrafiltration or dialysis method.

For a more accurate measure of free testosterone, use either equilibrium ultrafiltration or equilibrium dialysis. If neither of these options are available, then RIA can be used as a guide to follow changes in free testosterone. This is particularly important when working with an Ovarian Specialist to determine the correct dose of supplemental hormones to use to achieve a proper balance.

	RIA	Equilibrium Ultrafiltration	Equilibrium Dialysis
Range	0.3–3.2 pg/mL	1.0–8.5 pg/mL	1.0–8.5 pg/mL
Consistent	No	Yes	Yes

Table 6: Test methods for free testosterone

Another problem with laboratory reports is that there is no standard way of reporting the actual levels of hormone in the blood. Hormone levels are expressed as a concentration, and each laboratory decides which units they will use. Think of it this way: each laboratory has its own language that it speaks and it does not offer translation into any other language. Unfortunately it may be necessary to convert the results of your tests from unfamiliar units into units that are familiar to both you and your doctor. It goes without saying that if laboratories adopted one universal way of reporting hormone levels, converting results would not be necessary. However until that happens, it may be necessary to sharpen your math skills! Using all the same units to express ovarian hormone levels makes it much easier to see the relative amounts of each hormone. The following table reflects the levels of ovarian hormones if they were reported in the same units. As you can see in this example, there is 3 times more testosterone than estradiol, and 100 times more progesterone than estradiol! So, a tiny bit of estradiol goes a very long way.

Hormone	Current Method	Converted to Same Units
Estradiol	150 pg/ml	150 pg/ml
Testosterone	45 ng/ml	450 pg/ml
Progesterone	15 ng/ml	15,000 pg/ml

Table 7: Ovarian hormones expressed in the same units

It may be difficult at first to convert results; however it does get easier with practice. Table 8 is a reference table of some of the more common sets of units used to report levels of ovarian hormones.

Hormone	Measured In
Estradiol	picograms/milliliter (pg/ml) picomoles/Liter (pmol/L)
Testosterone	nanograms/deciliter (ng/dl) picomoles/Liter (pmol/L)
Progesterone	milligrams/milliliter (mg/ml) nanograms/milliliter (ng/ml)

Table 8: Reference table of different types of units used by laboratories

Key Points:
- Ovarian Specialists would address the gap in healthcare that currently exists for women
- The right lab test is important for accurate results, which means that you and your doctor need to understand your lab results to attain your goals

CHAPTER 8

SUMMING UP

Every organ in the body plays an important role on its own, and contributes to the well-being of every other organ. Should one, such as the ovaries, begin to fail, all others will be negatively affected. The ovaries, however, have always been thought of as "just" a reproductive organ. Instead of developing treatments to maintain or replace the function of the ovaries, women are encouraged to embrace ovarian failure. Then they're encouraged to live, however uncomfortably, with the fallout of that failure (which includes an increased risk for heart disease and breast cancer, osteoporosis, significant reduction in sexual functioning, and so on). We're told to eat right and exercise, and experience sexual encounters as if we still had functioning ovaries. This makes as much sense as expecting men who've suffered testicular failure to eat right and exercise and experience sexual encounters as if they still had functioning testes. It makes no sense for a man over the age of 50 to live out his life with testicular failure. So why do we say it makes sense for a woman of the same age to live out her life with ovarian failure? We're told that we should accept ovarian failure as a normal part of life. I believe that living with ovarian failure should be optional.

Other parts of our bodies have responded well to organ-extending treatment. For example, a hundred years ago no one would have expected a person's teeth to last much past the age of 30. We now recognize the benefits of early treatment, and start dental care on children as soon as they begin to get teeth. Today, this early and ongoing intervention allows all of us to expect our teeth to last a lifetime.

Other examples of organ-extending treatment include medications that have been developed to prevent heart disease, control high blood pressure, delay joint damage from arthritis, and prevent bone loss. The list is endless. Medical science has made tremendous contributions to our collective well-being. It is now important to extend this focus, and offer treatments to continue to improve the long-term well-being of women.

Normalizing ovarian function to extend the life of the ovary may significantly reduce breast cancer, colon cancer and heart disease, while sustaining sexual function and quality of sleep, and improving a woman's overall quality of life. Ovaries positively affect every organ system in a woman's body. Thus our focus should be to keep what works intact for as long as possible, and replace what's been lost as closely as possible after that. Normalizing ovarian function is no different than normalizing the function of any other organ in the body. We don't think twice about taking medication to improve the function of our kidneys, heart or eyes. Why then not seek treatment for our ovaries, too?

We have accepted an unacceptable situation for too long, and it is definitely time for a change. You can be a part of this change. Ask your doctor or healthcare professional for help. Together, we can insist on better information, better testing and better products. Our health and happiness depends on it.

MY JOURNEY CONTINUES

I am very fortunate. I found the answers I was looking for. I now know that maintaining the ovarian hormone balance that once was achieved by my ovaries is my responsibility, and I am healthier for it. I believe I have significantly reduced my risk for breast cancer, heart disease and osteoporosis. I have mostly restored my sexual function. Until more versatile hormone products are available, I will continue to struggle to find *my* right balance. At times I am overwhelmed by the complexity of replacing the function of my ovaries, and at other times appreciate that I can even try. I look forward to a day when effective, convenient and affordable products are available.

I can think clearly again. I have my life back now. It is woven with a deep appreciation of what was lost and what has been regained.

THE FUTURE OF MENOPAUSE ... FOR OURSELVES, OUR DAUGHTERS AND OUR GRANDDAUGHTERS

Having read this book, you know that the culture for the next generation of menopausal women is changing. University teaching hospitals can create a more appropriate curriculum for an Ovarian Specialist. Pharmaceutical companies can be lobbied to create more appropriate therapies. For more information about advocacy work in this area, visit my website: *www.PreventingMenopause.com.*

May the future be better for ourselves, our daughters and our granddaughters.

CHECKLIST

1) Find the right healthcare provider. The right provider:
    a. Is committed to your goal of preventing menopause.
    b. Understands the interactions of the various ovarian hormones.

2) Determine how many years of ovarian function you have left without further treatment. Find your levels of:
    a. FSH
    b. LH
    c. Total Estradiol
    d. Total Testosterone
    e. Free Testosterone
    f. Progesterone
    g. SHBG
    h. Inhibin B

3) Determine the date that your ovaries are calculated to fail. You will need an ultrasound to determine the volume of your ovaries. From this volume your doctor can calculate what age your ovaries will fail.[1]

4) Determine whether or not you need to supplement inhibin and/or testosterone. Normal levels can be found in Table 3: "Recommended hormone levels prior to ovarian failure."
    a. Once inhibin and testosterone are at normal levels the ovary can produce normal levels of estradiol and progesterone.
    b. Check FSH on days 3 to 5 of your menstrual cycle and track your progress.

5) To maintain optimal ovarian function it will be important to do the following:

   a. Exercise regularly. Exercise helps to maintain consistent hormone levels.

   b. Avoid medications and substances that can change the levels of ovarian hormones, either directly or by increasing SHBG (see page 25: "How All Hormones Are Stored in the Blood").

   c. Read the labels on all your medications. Any medicine that causes impotence in a man will cause sexual problems in a woman! Any substance that is toxic to the testes will be toxic to the ovaries.

   d. Have a frank talk with your doctor and pharmacist. Insist on knowing if the binding proteins for estradiol and testosterone, SHBG, and for progesterone, CBG, will not change substantially with a particular medication. If they do not know, then insist they find out! If they refuse, then it is time to find a new doctor and pharmacist.

6) Re-do all four hormone tests—estradiol, testosterone (free and total), FSH and inhibin—to see that they are all in a reasonable range.

7) Have a yearly ultrasound to track your progress and to ensure that your ovaries are not being depleted of eggs too soon!

	GOALS	Date			
FSH Day 3					
LH					
Total Estradiol					
Total Testosterone					
Free Testosterone					
Progesterone					
SHBG					
Inhibin B					
Ovarian Volume/ Calculated Date of Exhaustion					

RESOURCES

Finding a Doctor Who Can Help You

Once you have decided on your goals you will need to find a doctor or other healthcare professional with whom to work. While many women work with a gynecologist, it is just as valid to work with an endocrinologist, internist, family practitioner or any other type of healthcare professional that is open to new ideas and is willing to work with you. Also, even if your doctor is eager to work with you he or she may be new to prescribing hormones. But if you work together with patience and a common goal, you *can* get there. Share your copy of my book with your healthcare professional, and embark together on a journey to improve and maintain your ovarian health.

To see what you can do to help the medical and pharmaceutical industries understand that more information and better products are needed, visit my website: *www.PreventingMenopause.com.*

BIBLIOGRAPHY

1. Changing the Way We Think

1. O'Connor K.A., Holman D.J., Wood J.W. "Menstrual cycle variability and the perimenopause." *Am J Human Biol.* 13(4): 465-78, Jul-Aug 2001.

2. Dimitrakakis C., Zhou J., Wang J., Belanger A., LaBrie F., Cheng C., Powell D., Bondy C. "A physiologic role for testosterone in limiting estrogenic stimulation of the breast." *Menopause.* 10(4): 292-8, Jul-Aug 2003.

3. Zhou J., Ng S., Adesanya-Famuiya O., Anderson K., Bondy C.A. "Testosterone inhibits estrogen-induced mammary epithelial proliferation and suppresses estrogen receptor expression." *FASEB J.* 14(12): 1725-30, Sep 2000.

2. A Common Language and a Common Goal

1. Chryssikopoulos A. "The potential role of intraovarian factors on ovarian androgen production." *Ann N Y Acad Sci.* 900: 184-92, 2000.

2. [No authors listed] "Design of the Women's Health Initiative clinical trial and observational study; The Women's Health Initiative Study Group." *Control Clin Trials.* 19(1): 61-109, Feb 2000.

3. "Cancer Facts & Figures 2004." Retrieved online at: http://www.cancer.org/downloads/STT/CAF2004PWSecured.pdf, June 29 2004.

4. Robertson A.K., Rudling M., Zhou X., Gorelik L., Flavell R.A., Hansson G.K. "Disruption of TGF-beta signaling in T cells accelerates atherosclerosis." *J Clin Invest.* 112(9): 1342-50, Nov 2003.

5. Mercuro G., Zoncu S., Saiu F., Mascia M., Melis G.B., Rosano G.M. "Menopause induced by oophorectomy reveals a role of ovarian estrogen on the maintenance of pressure homeostasis." *Maturitas.* 47(2): 131-8, Feb 20 2004.

6. Rosano G.M., Leonardo F., Dicandia C., Sheiban I., Pagnotta P., Pappone C., Chierchia S.L. "Acute electrophysiologic effect of estradiol 17beta in menopausal women." *Am J Cardiol.* 86(12): 1385-7, A5-6, Dec 15 2000.

7. Ben Aryeh H., Gottlieb I., Ish-Shalom S., David A., Szargel H., Laufer D. "Oral complaints related to menopause." *Maturitas.* 24(3): 185-9, Jul 1996.

8. Reddy M.S. "Oral osteoporosis: is there an association between periodontitis and osteoporosis?" *Compend Contin Educ Dent.* 23(10 Suppl): 21-8, Oct 2002

9. Bolognia J.L., Braverman I.M., Rousseau M.E., Sarrel P.M. "Skin changes in menopause." *Maturitas.* 11(4): 295-304, Dec 1989.

10. Sherwin B.B. "Estrogen effects on cognition in menopausal women." *Neurology.* 48(5 Suppl 7): S21-6, May 1997.

11. Connell K., Guess M.K., Bleustein C.B., Powers K., Lazarou G., Mikhail M., Melman A. "Effects of age, menopause, and comorbidities on neurological function of the female genitalia." *Int J Impot Res.* May 27 2004.

12. Berman J.R., Berman L.A., Werbin T.J., Flaherty E.E., Leahy N.M., Goldstein I. "Clinical evaluation of female sexual function: effects of age and estrogen status on subjective and physiologic sexual responses." *Int J Impot Res.* 11 Suppl 1: S31-8, Sep 1999.

13. Triadafilopoulos G., Finlayson M., Grellet C. "Bowel dysfunction in postmenopausal women." *Women Health.* 27(4): 55-66. 1998.

14. Reddy M.S. "Oral osteoporosis: is there an association between periodontitis and osteoporosis?" *Compend Contin Educ Dent.* 23(10 Suppl): 21-8, Oct 2002.

15. Macdonald H.M., New S.A., Campbell M.K., Reid D.M. "Longitudinal changes in weight in perimenopausal and early postmenopausal women: effects of dietary energy intake, energy expenditure, dietary calcium intake and hormone replacement therapy." *Int J Obes Relat Metab Disord.* 27(6): 669-76, Jun 2003.

16. Toth M.J., Tchernof A., Sites C.K., Poehlman E.T. "Effect of menopausal status on body composition and abdominal fat distribution." *Int J Obes Relat Metab Disord.* 24(2): 226-31, Feb 2000.

17. Platen P. Hoffmann L., Schiffman D., Diel P. "mRNA Expression of Estrogen Receptor (ER), Progesterone Receptor (PR) and cFOS in Skeletal Muscle in Female Athletes in Different Phases of their Menstrual Cycle." Retrieved online at: http://www.thieme.de/abstracts/eced/abstracts2002/daten/v036.html. June 28 2004.

18. Wiik A., Glenmark B., Ekman M., Esbjornsson-Liljedahl M., Johansson O., Bodin K., Enmark E., Jansson E. "Oestrogen receptor beta is expressed in adult human skeletal muscle both at the mRNA and protein level." *Acta Physiol Scand.* 79(4): 381-7, Dec 2003.

19. Bixler E.O., Vgontzas A.N., Lin H.M., Ten Have T., Rein J., Vela-Bueno A., Kales A. "Prevalence of sleep-disordered breathing in women: effects of gender." *Am J Respir Crit Care Med.* 163(3 Pt 1): 608-13, Mar 2001.

20. Netzer N.C., Eliasson A.H., Strohl K.P. 'Women with sleep apnea have lower levels of sex hormones." *Sleep Breath.* 7(1): 25-9, Mar 2003.

21. National Sleep Foundation. "Women & Sleep: Most Common Sleep Problems in Women." Retrieved online at: http://www.sleepfoundation.org/publications/women.cfm. June 28 2004.

22. Saad Z., Vincent M., Bramwell V., Stitt L., Duff J., Girotti M., Jory T., Heathcote G., Turnbull I., Garcia B. "Timing of surgery influences survival in receptor-negative as well as receptor-positive breast cancer." *Eur J Cancer.* 30A(9): 1348-52, 1994.

23. Formenti S., Felix J., Salonga D., Danenberg K., Pike M.C., Danenberg P. "Expression of metastases-associated genes in cervical cancers resected in the proliferative and secretory phases of the menstrual cycle." *Clin Cancer Res.* 6(12): 4653-7, Dec 2000.

24. Lutgens E., Gijbels M., Smook M., Heeringa P., Gotwals P., Kotelian-sky V.E., Daemen M.J. "Transforming growth factor-beta mediates balance between inflammation and fibrosis during plaque progression." *Arterioscler Thromb Vasc Biol.* 22(6): 975-82, Jun 1 2002.

25. Mallat Z., Gojova A., Marchiol-Fournigault C., Esposito B., Kamate C., Merval R., Fradelizi D., Tedgui A. "Inhibition of transforming growth factor-beta signaling accelerates atherosclerosis and induces an unstable plaque phenotype in mice." *Circ Res.* 89(10): 930-4, Nov 9 2001.

26. Robertson A.K., Rudling M., Zhou X., Gorelik L., Flavell R.A., Hansson G.K. "Disruption of TGF-beta signaling in T cells accelerates atherosclerosis." *J Clin Invest.* 112(9):1342-50, Nov 2003.

3. Why Prevent Ovarian Failure?

1. Diamond, Jared, Ph.D. *Why Is Sex Fun?: The Evolution of Human Sexuality.* New York: Basic Books (1998).

2. Somboonporn W., Davis S.R. "Postmenopausal testosterone therapy and breast cancer risk." *Maturitas.* 49(4): 267-75, Dec 10 2004.

3. Rosenthal, M.S., Ph.D. *The Fertility Sourcebook.* New York: McGraw-Hill (2002).

4. Bachmann G., Bancroft J., Braunstein G., Burger H., Davis S., Dennerstein L., Goldstein I., Guay A., Leiblum S., Lobo R., Notelovitz M., Rosen R., Sarrel P., Sherwin B., Simon J., Simpson E., Shifren J, Spark R., Traish A., Princeton "Female androgen insufficiency: the Princeton consensus statement on definition, classification, and assessment." *Fertil Steril.* 77(4): 660-5, Apr 2002.

5. Labrie F., Luu-The V., Labrie C., Belanger A., Simard J., Lin S.X., Pelletier G. "Endocrine and intracrine sources of androgens in women: inhibition of breast cancer and other roles of androgens and their precursor dehydroepiandrosterone." *Endocr Rev.* 24(2): 152-82, Apr 2003.

6. Shaaban A.M., O'Neill P.A., Davies M.P., Sibson R., West C.R., Smith P.H., Foster C.S. "Declining estrogen receptor-beta expression defines malignant progression of human breast neoplasia." *Am J Surg Pathol.* 27(12):1502-12, Dec 2003.

7. Dimitrakakis C., Zhou J., Bondy C.A. "Androgens and mammary growth and neoplasia." *Fertil Steril.* 77 Suppl 4: S26-33, Apr 2002.

8. Dimitrakakis C., Zhou J., Wang J., Belanger A., LaBrie F., Cheng C., Powell D., Bondy C. "A physiologic role for testosterone in limiting estrogenic stimulation of the breast." *Menopause.* 10(4): 292-8, Jul-Aug 2003.

9. Lawson J.S., Field A.S., Tran D.D., Houssami N. "Hormone replacement therapy use dramatically increases breast oestrogen receptor expression in obese postmenopausal women." *Breast Cancer Res.* 3(5): 342-5, 2001.

10. Paruthiyil S., Parmar H., Kerekatte V., Cunha G.R., Firestone G.L., Leitman D.C. "Estrogen receptor beta inhibits human breast cancer cell proliferation and tumor formation by causing a G2 cell cycle arrest." *Cancer Res.* 64(1): 423-8, Jan 1 2004.

11. Zhou J., Ng S., Adesanya-Famuiya O., Anderson K., Bondy C.A. "Testosterone inhibits estrogen-induced mammary epithelial proliferation and suppresses estrogen receptor expression." *FASEB J.* 14(12): 1725-30, Sep 2000.

12. Giordano S.H., Buzdar A.U., Hortobagyi G.N. "Breast cancer in men." *Ann Intern Med.* 137(8): 678-87, Oct 15 2002.

13. Anderson W.F., Althuis M.D., Brinton L.A., Devesa S.S. "Is male breast cancer similar or different than female breast cancer?" *Breast Cancer Res Treat.* 83(1): 77-86, Jan 2004.

14. Pathology Associates Medical Laboratories. "ESTRADIOl." Retrieved online at: http://etd.paml.com/etd/display.php?ordercode=ESTRADIOAL &and=&andand. June 21 2004.

15. Laboratory Corporation of America. "Estradiol, Sensitive." Retrieved online at: http://www.labcorp.com/datasets/labcorp/html/chapter/mono/ sr012000. June 21 2004.

16. American Cancer Society. "Breast Cancer Facts & Figures 2001-2002."

17. Lau K.M., Mok S.C., Ho S.M. "Expression of human estrogen receptor-alpha and -beta, progesterone receptor, and androgen receptor mRNA in normal and malignant ovarian epithelial cells." *Proc Natl Acad Sci U S A.* 96(10): 5722-7, May 11 1999.

18. Sakaguchi H., Fujimoto J., Aoki I., Tamaya T. "Expression of estrogen receptor alpha and beta in myometrium of premenopausal and postmenopausal women." *Steroids.* 68(1): 11-9, Jan 2003.

19. Sakaguchi H., Fujimoto J., Aoki I., Toyoki H., Khatun S., Tamaya T. "Expression of oestrogen receptor alpha and beta in uterine endometrial and ovarian cancers." *Eur J Cancer.* 38 Suppl 6: S74-5, Nov 2002.

20. Fujimoto J., Hirose R., Sakaguchi H., Tamaya T. "Clinical significance of expression of estrogen receptor alpha and beta mRNAs in ovarian cancers." *Oncology.* 58(4): 334-41, May 2000.

21. Lerner D.J., Kannel W.B. "Patterns of coronary heart disease morbidity and mortality in the sexes: a 26-year follow-up of the Framingham population." *Am Heart J.* 111(2): 383-90, Feb 1986; *Int J Sports Med.* 23(7): 477-83, Oct 1986.

22. Lawler J.M., Hu Z., Green J.S., Crouse S.F., Grandjean P.W., Bounds R.G. "Combination of estrogen replacement and exercise protects against HDL oxidation in post-menopausal women." 2002.

23. Gong M., Wilson M., Kelly T., Su W., Dressman J., Kincer J., Matveev S.V., Guo L., Guerin T., Li X.A., Zhu W., Uittenbogaard A., Smart E.J. "HDL-associated estradiol stimulates endothelial NO synthase and vasodilation in an SR-BI-dependent manner." *J Clin Invest.* 111(10): 1579-87, May 2003.

24. Abplanalp W., Scheiber M.D., Moon K., Kessel B., Liu J.H., Subbiah M.T. "Evidence for the role of high density lipoproteins in mediating the antioxidant effect of estrogens." *Eur J Endocrinol.* 142(1): 79-83, Jan 2000.

25. Tang M., Abplanalp W., Subbiah M.T. "Association of estrogens with human plasma lipoproteins: studies using estradiol-17beta and its hydrophobic derivative". *J Lab Clin Med.* 129(4): 447-52, Apr 1997.

26. Mercuro G., Zoncu S., Saiu F., Mascia M., Melis G.B., Rosano G.M. "Menopause induced by oophorectomy reveals a role of ovarian estrogen on the maintenance of pressure homeostasis." *Maturitas.* 47(2): 131-8, Feb 20 2004.

27. Vongpatanasin W., Tuncel M., Mansour Y., Arbique D., Victor R.G. "Transdermal estrogen replacement therapy decreases sympathetic activity in postmenopausal women." *Circulation.* 103(24): 2903-8, Jun 19 2001.

28. Brideau N.A., Forest J.C., Lemay A., Dodin S. "Correlation between ovarian steroids and lipid fractions in relation to age in premenopausal women." *Clin Endocrinol* (Oxf). 37(5): 437-44, Nov 1992.

29. Chu M.C., Rath K.M., Huie J., Taylor H.S. "Elevated basal FSH in normal cycling women is associated with unfavourable lipid levels and increased cardiovascular risk." *Hum Reprod.* 18(8):1570-3, Aug 2003.

30. National Sleep Foundation. "Women & Sleep, Insomnia." Retrieved online at: http://www.sleepfoundation.org/publications/women.cfm. June 28 2004.

31. National Sleep Foundation. "Women & Sleep,Melatonin." Retrieved online at: http://www.sleepfoundation.org/publications/women.cfm. June 28 2004.

32. Montplaisir J., Lorrain J., Denesle R., Petit D., "Sleep in menopause: differential effects of two forms of hormone replacement therapy." *Menopause.* 8(1): 10-6, Jan-Feb 2001.

33. Zoccoli G., Grant D.A., Wild J., Walker A.M. "Nitric oxide inhibition abolishes sleep-wake differences in cerebral circulation." *Am J Physiol Heart Circ Physiol.* 280(6): H2598-606, Jun 2001.

34. National Sleep Foundation. "Women & Sleep, Understanding Your Monthly Cycle." Retrieved online at: http://www.sleepfoundation.org/publications/women.cfm. June 28 2004.

35. Cagnacci A., Arangino S., Angiolucci M., Melis G.B., Facchinetti F., Malmusi S., Volpe A. "Effect of exogenous melatonin on vascular reactivity and nitric oxide in postmenopausal women: role of hormone replacement therapy." *Clin Endocrinol* (Oxf). 54(2): 261-6, Feb 2001.

36. Macdonald H.M., New S.A., Campbell M.K., Reid D.M. "Longitudinal changes in weight in perimenopausal and early postmenopausal women: effects of dietary energy intake, energy expenditure, dietary calcium intake and hormone replacement therapy." *Int J Obes Relat Metab Disord.* 27(6): 669-76, Jun 2003.

37. Toth M.J., Tchernof A., Sites C.K., Poehlman E.T. "Effect of menopausal status on body composition and abdominal fat distribution." *Int J Obes Relat Metab Disord.* 24(2): 226-31, Feb 2000.

38. Belanger C., Luu-The V., Dupont P., Tchernof A. "Adipose tissue intracrinology: potential importance of local androgen/estrogen metabolism in the regulation of adiposity." *Horm Metab Res.* 34(11-12): 737-45, Nov-Dec 2002.

39. Heiss C.J., Sanborn C.F., Nichols D.L., Bonnick S.L., Alford B.B. "Associations of body fat distribution, circulating sex hormones, and bone density in postmenopausal women." *J Clin Endocrinol Metab.* 80(5): 1591-6, May 1995.

40. Wiik A., Glenmark B., Ekman M., Esbjornsson-Liljedahl M., Johansson O., Bodin K., Enmark E., Jansson E. "Oestrogen receptor beta is expressed in adult human skeletal muscle both at the mRNA and protein level." *Acta Physiol Scand.* 179(4): 381-7, Dec 2003.

41. Berman J.R., Berman L.A., Werbin T.J., Flaherty E.E., Leahy N.M., Goldstein I. "Clinical evaluation of female sexual function: effects of age and estrogen status on subjective and physiologic sexual responses." *Int J Impot Res.*11 Suppl 1: S31-8, Sep 1999.

42. Warnock J.K., Bundren J.C., Morris D.W. "Female hypoactive sexual disorder: case studies of physiologic androgen replacement." *J Sex Marital Ther.* 25(3): 175-82, Jul-Sep 1999.

43. Thompson C.A., Shanafelt T.D., Loprinzi C.L. "Andropause: symptom management for prostate cancer patients treated with hormonal ablation." *Oncologist.* 8(5):474-87, 2003.

4. How To Prevent Ovarian Failure

1. Orentreich N., Brind J.L., Rizer R.L., Vogelman J.H. "Age changes and sex differences in serum dehydroepiandrosterone sulfate concentrations throughout adulthood." *J Clin Endocrinol Metab.* 59(3): 551-5, Sep 1984.

2. MacNaughton J., Banah M., McCloud P., Hee J., Burger H. "Age related changes in follicle stimulating hormone, luteinizing hormone, oestradiol and immunoreactive inhibin in women of reproductive age." *Clin Endocrinol* (Oxf). 36(4): 339-45, Apr 1992.

3. Eagleson C.A., Gingrich M.B., Pastor C.L., Arora T.K., Burt C.M., Evans W.S., Marshall J.C. "Polycystic ovarian syndrome: evidence that flutamide restores sensitivity of the gonadotropin-releasing hormone pulse generator to inhibition by estradiol and progesterone." *J Clin Endocrinol Metab.* 85(11): 4047-52, Nov 2000.

4. Faddy M.J. "Follicle dynamics during ovarian ageing." *Mol Cell Endocrinol.* 163(1-2): 43-8, May 25 2000.

5. Gosden R.G., Faddy M.J. "Ovarian aging, follicular depletion, and steroidogenesis." *Exp Gerontol.* 29(3-4): 265-74, May-Aug 1994.

6. Faddy M.J., Gosden R.G. "A mathematical model of follicle dynamics in the human ovary." *Hum Reprod.* 10(4): 770-5, Apr 1995.

7. Cramer D.W., Xu H., Harlow B.L. "Does "incessant" ovulation increase risk for early menopause?" *Am J Obstet Gynecol.* 172(2 Pt 1): 568-73, Feb 1995.

8. Ozawa M., Shi F., Watanabe G., Suzuki A.K., Taya K. "Regulatory role of inhibin in follicle-stimulating hormone secretion and folliculogenesis in the guinea pig." *J Vet Med Sci.* 63(10):1091-5, Oct 2001.

9. Gougeon A., Ecochard R., Thalabard J.C. "Age-related changes of the population of human ovarian follicles: increase in the disappearance rate of non-growing and early-growing follicles in aging women." *Biol Reprod.* 50(3): 653-63, Mar 1994.

10. Erickson, Gregory F. *Menopause, Biology and Pathobiology.* "Chapter 2: Ovarian Anatomy and Physiology (13-32)." San Diego: Academic Press (2001).

11. Lee S.J., Lenton E.A., Sexton L., Cooke I.D. "The effect of age on the cyclical patterns of plasma LH, FSH, oestradiol and progesterone in women with regular menstrual cycles." *Hum Reprod.* 3(7): 851-5, Oct 1998.

12. Sodergard R., Backstrom T., Shanbhag V., Carstensen H. "Calculation of free and bound fractions of testosterone and estradiol-17 beta to human plasma proteins at body temperature." *J Steroid Biochem.* 16(6):801-, Jun 1982.

13. Minassian S.S., Wu C.H. "Free and protein-bound progesterone during normal and luteal phase defective cycles." *Int J Gynaecol Obstet.* 43(2): 163-8, Nov 1993.

14. Longcope C., Hui S.L., Johnston C.C. Jr. "Free estradiol, free testosterone, and sex hormone-binding globulin in perimenopausal women." *J Clin Endocrinol Metab.* 64(3): 513-8, Mar 1987.

15. Vincens M., Mercier-Bodard C., Mowszowicz I., Kuttenn F., Mauvais-Jarvis P. "Testosterone-estradiol binding globulin (TeBG) in hirsute patients treated with cyproterone acetate (CPA) and percutaneous estradiol." *J Steroid Biochem.* 33(4A):531-4, Oct 1998.

16. Hammond G.L., Nisker J.A., Jones L.A., Siiteri P.K. "Estimation of the percentage of free steroid in undiluted serum by centrifugal ultrafiltration-dialysis." *J Biol Chem.* 255(11): 5023-6, Jun 10 1980.

17. Moll G.W. Jr., Rosenfield R.L. "Plasma free testosterone in the diagnosis of adolescent polycystic ovary syndrome." *J Pediatr.* 102(3): 461-4, Mar 1983.

18. Mean F., Pellaton M., Magrini G. "Study on the binding of dihydrotes-tosterone, testosterone and oestradiol with sex hormone binding globulin." *Clin Chim Acta.* 80(1): 171-80, Oct 1 1977.

19. Labrie F., Belanger A., Cusan L., Gomez J.L., Candas B. "Marked decline in serum concentrations of adrenal C19 sex steroid precursors and conju-gated androgen metabolites during aging." *J Clin Endocrinol Metab.* 82(8): 2396-402, Aug 1997.

20. Santoro N., Isaac B., Neal-Perry G., Adel T., Weingart L., Nussbaum A., Thakur S., Jinnai H., Khosla N., Barad D. "Impaired folliculogenesis and ovulation in older reproductive aged women." *J Clin Endocrinol Metab.* 88(11): 5502-9, Nov 2003.

21. Carcio, H.A. *Management of the Infertile Woman.* Philadelphia :Lippin-cott-Raven Publishers (1998).

22. Weil S., Vendola K., Zhou J., Bondy C.A. "Androgen and follicle-stimu-lating hormone interactions in primate ovarian follicle development." *J Clin Endocrinol Metab.* 84(8): 2951-6, Aug 1999.

23. Vendola K.A., Zhou J., Adesanya O.O., Weil S.J., Bondy C.A. "Andro-gens stimulate early stages of follicular growth in the primate ovary." *J Clin Invest.* 101(12): 2622-9, Jun 15 1998.

24. Wang P.H., Chang C. "Androgens and ovarian cancers." *Eur J Gynaecol Oncol.* 25(2): 157-63, Jun 15 1998.

25. Sheth A.R., Vijayalakshmi S. "Selective suppression of FSH as a possible approach for fertility regulation." *Arch Androl.* 7(2): 109-15, Sep 1981.

26. de Vries E., den Tonkelaar I., van Noord P.A., van der Schouw Y.T., te Velde E.R., Peeters P.H. "Oral contraceptive use in relation to age at meno-pause in the DOM cohort." *Hum Reprod.* 16(8): 1657-62, Aug 2001.

27. Keizer H.A., Kuipers H., Verstappen F.T., Janssen E. "Limitations of concentration measurements for evaluation of endocrine status of exercising women." *Can J Appl Sport Sci.* 7(2): 79-84, Jun 1982.

28. Lucero J., Harlow B.L., Barbieri R.L., Sluss P., Cramer D.W. "Early fol-licular phase hormone levels in relation to patterns of alcohol, tobacco, and coffee use." *Fertil Steril.* 76(4): 723-9, Oct 2001.

29. Hardy R., Kuh D., Wadsworth M. "Smoking, body mass index, socioeconomic status and the menopausal transition in a British national cohort." *Int J Epidemiol.* 29(5): 845-51, Oct 2001.

30. Daniel M., Martin A.D., Faiman C. "Sex hormones and adipose tissue distribution in premenopausal cigarette smokers." *Int J Obes Relat Metab Disord.* 16(4): 245-54, Apr 1992.

31. Pugeat M.M., Dunn J.F., Nisula B.C. "Transport of steroid hormones: interaction of 70 drugs with testosterone-binding globulin and corticosteroid-binding globulin in human plasma." *J Clin Endocrinol Metab.* 53(1): 69-75, Jul 1981.

32. Pereyra Pacheco B., Mendez Ribas J.M., Milone G., Fernandez I., Kvicala R., Mila T., Di Noto A., Contreras Ortiz O., Pavlovsky S. "Use of GnRH analogs for functional protection of the ovary and preservation of fertility during cancer treatment in adolescents: a preliminary report." *Gynecol Oncol.* 81(3): 391-7, Jun 2001.

33. Recchia F., Sica G., De Filippis S., Saggio G., Rosselli M., Rea S. "Goserelin as ovarian protection in the adjuvant treatment of premenopausal breast cancer: a phase II pilot study." *Anticancer Drugs.* 13(4): 417-24, Apr 2002.

34. Meirow D., Epstein M., Lewis H., Nugent D., Gosden R.G. "Administration of cyclophosphamide at different stages of follicular maturation in mice: effects on reproductive performance and fetal malformations." *Hum Reprod.* 16(4): 632-7, Apr 2001.

35. Meirow D., Lewis H., Nugent D., Epstein M. "Subclinical depletion of primordial follicular reserve in mice treated with cyclophosphamide: clinical importance and proposed accurate investigative tool." *Hum Reprod.* 14(7): 1903-7, Jul 2001.

36. Van Thiel D.H., Gavaler J.S., Lester R., Goodman M.D. "Alcohol-induced testicular atrophy. An experimental model for hypogonadism occurring in chronic alcoholic men." *Gastroenterology.* 69(2): 326-32, Aug 1975.

37. Van Thiel D.H., Gavaler J.S., Eagon P.K., Chiao Y.B., Cobb C.F., Lester R. "Alcohol and sexual function." *Pharmacol Biochem Behav.* 13 Suppl 1:125-9, 1980.

5. Restoring the Balance

1. Piltonen T., Koivunen R., Ruokonen A., Tapanainen J.S. "Ovarian age-related responsiveness to human chorionic gonadotropin." *J Clin Endocrinol Metab.* 88(7): 3327-32, Jul 2003.

2. Cowan L.D., Gordis L., Tonascia J.A., Jones G.S. "Breast cancer incidence in women with a history of progesterone deficiency." *Am J Epidemiol.* 114(2): 209-17, Aug 1981.

3. Davidson B.J., Ross R.K., Paganini-Hill A., Hammond G.D., Siiteri P.K., Judd H.L. "Total and free estrogens and androgens in postmenopausal women with hip fractures." *J Clin Endocrinol Metab.* 54(1): 115-20, Jan 1982.

4. Schiavone F.E., Rietschel R.L., Sgoutas D., Harris R. "Elevated free testosterone levels in women with acne." *Arch Dermatol.* 119(10): 799-802, Oct 1983.

5. Serin I.S., Ozcelik B., Basbug M., Aygen E., Kula M., Erez R. "Long-term effects of continuous oral and transdermal estrogen replacement therapy on sex hormone binding globulin and free testosterone levels." *Eur J Obstet Gynecol Reprod Biol.* 99(2): 222-5, Dec 1 2001.

6. Vihtamaki T., Tuimala R. "Can climacteric women self-adjust therapeutic estrogen doses using symptoms as markers?" *Maturitas.* 28(3): 199-203, Jan 12 1998.

7. Estrasorb. "Novavax, Prescribing Information." 2004.

8. Dodson K.S., Coutts J.R., MacNaughton M.C. "Plasma sex steroid and gonadotrophin patterns in human menstrual cycles." *Br J Obstet Gynaecol.* 82(8): 602-14, Aug 1975.

9. Simon J.A., Robinson D.E., Andrews M.C., Hildebrand J.R. 3rd, Rocci M.L. Jr., Blake R.E., Hodgen G.D. "The absorption of oral micronized progesterone: the effect of food, dose proportionality, and comparison with intramuscular progesterone." *Fertil Steril.* 60(1): 26-33, Jul 1993.

10. Wallace W.H., Kelsey T.W. "Ovarian reserve and reproductive age may be determined from measurement of ovarian volume by transvaginal sonography." *Hum Reprod.* Jun 17 2004.

11. Sheth A.R., Vijayalakshmi S. "Selective suppression of FSH as a possible approach for fertility regulation." *Arch Androl.* 7(2): 109-15, Sep 1981.

6. Understanding Standard Hormore Replacement Therapy as Used in the Women's Health Initiative

1. [No authors listed] "Design of the Women's Health Initiative clinical trial and observational study. The Women's Health Initiative Study Group." *Control Clin Trials.* 19(1): 61-109, Feb 1998.

2. Nachtigall L.E., Raju U., Banerjee S., Wan L., Levitz M. "Serum estradiol-binding profiles in postmenopausal women undergoing three common estrogen replacement therapies: associations with sex hormone-binding globulin, estradiol, and estrone levels." *Menopause.* 7(4): 243-50, Jul-Aug 2000.

3. Yasui T., Uemura H., Tezuka M., Yamada M., Irahara M., Miura M., Aono T. "Biological effects of hormone replacement therapy in relation to serum estradiol levels." *Horm Res.* 56(1-2): 38-44, 2001.

4. Sodergard R., Backstrom T., Shanbhag V., Carstensen H. "Calculation of free and bound fractions of testosterone and estradiol-17 beta to human plasma proteins at body temperature." *J Steroid Biochem.* 16(6): 801-10, Jun 1982.

5. Minassian S.S., Wu C.H. "Free and protein-bound progesterone during normal and luteal phase defective cycles." *Int J Gynaecol Obstet.* 43(2): 163-8, Nov 1993.

6. Vongpatanasin W. Tuncel M., Wang Z., Arbique D., Mehrad B., Jialal I. "Differential effects of oral versus transdermal estrogen replacement therapy on C-reactive protein in postmenopausal women." *J Am Coll Cardiol.* 41(8): 1358-63, Apr 16 2003.

7. Arafah B.M. "Increased need for thyroxine in women with hypothyroidism during estrogen therapy." *N Engl J Med.* 344(23): 1743-9, Jun 7 2001.

8. Sowers M., Luborsky J., Perdue C., Araujo K.L., Goldman M.B., Harlow S.D. SWAN. "Thyroid stimulating hormone (TSH) concentrations and menopausal status in women at the mid-life: SWAN." *Clin Endocrinol* (Oxf). 58(3): 340-7, Mar 2003.

9. Vihtamaki T., Savilahti R., Tuimala R. "Why do postmenopausal women discontinue hormone replacement therapy?" *Maturitas.* 33(2): 99-105, Oct 24 1999.

10. Adams M.R., Register T.C., Golden D.L., Wagner J.D., Williams J.K. "Medroxyprogesterone acetate antagonizes inhibitory effects of conjugated equine estrogens on coronary artery atherosclerosis." *Arterioscler Thromb Vasc Biol.* 17(1): 217-21, Jan 1997.

11. Fraser I.S. "Plasma lipid changes and medroxyprogesterone acetate." *Contracept Deliv Syst.* 4(1): 1-7, Jan 1983.

12. Gordon G.G., Southren A.L., Tochimoto S., Olivo J., Altman K., Rand J., Lemberger L. "Effect of medroxyprogesterone acetate (Provera) on the metabolism and biological activity of testosterone." *J Clin Endocrinol Metab.* 30(4): 449-56, Apr 1970.

13. Gordon G.G., Altman K., Southren A.L., Olivo J. "Human hepatic testosterone A-ring reductase activity: effect of medroxyprogesterone acetate." *J Clin Endocrinol Metab.* 32(4): 457-61, Apr 1971.

14. Miyagawa K., Rosch J., Stanczyk F., Hermsmeyer K. "Medroxyprogesterone interferes with ovarian steroid protection against coronary vasospasm." *Nat Med.* 3(3): 324-7, Mar 1997.

15. Minshall R.D., Stanczyk F.Z., Miyagawa K., Uchida B., Axthelm M., Novy M., Hermsmeyer K. "Ovarian steroid protection against coronary artery hyperreactivity in rhesus monkeys." *J Clin Endocrinol Metab.* 83(2): 649-59, Feb 1998.

16. Wyeth. "Premarin-conjugated equine estrogen tablets prescribing information." Retrieved online at:http://www.wyeth.com/content/ShowLabeling. asp?id=131. June 20 2004.

7. Working with Your Medical Professional

1. Gruschke A., Kuhl H. "Validity of radioimmunological methods for determining free testosterone in serum." *Fertil Steril.* 76(3): 576-82, Sep 2001.

2. Rosner W. "An extraordinarily inaccurate assay for free testosterone is still with us." *J Clin Endocrinol Metab.* 86(6): 2903, Jun 2001.

3. Sinha-Hikim I., Arver S., Beall G., Shen R., Guerrero M., Sattler F., Shikuma C., Nelson J.C., Landgren B.M., Mazer N.A., Bhasin S. "The use of a sensitive equilibrium dialysis method for the measurement of free testosterone levels in healthy, cycling women and in human immunodeficiency virus-

infected women." *J Clin Endocrinol Metab.* 83(4): 1312-8, Apr 1998.

4. Vermeulen A., Verdonck L,. Kaufman J.M. "A critical evaluation of simple methods for the estimation of free testosterone in serum." *J Clin Endocrinol Metab.* 84(10): 3666-72, Oct 1999.

5. Esoterix, Inc Laboratory Services. "TESTOSTERONE, FREE, BLOOD (INCLUDES TOTAL)." Retrieved online at: http://webserver01.bjc.org/labtestguide/TestostFree.htm. June 19 2004.

6. Laboratory Corporation of America. "Testosterone (Free), Serum (by Equilibrium Ultrafiltration) With Total Testosterone." Retrieved online at: http://www.labcorp.com/datasets/labcorp/html/chapter/mono/sr003800.htm. June 19 2004.

7. Diagnostics Systems Laboratory Inc. "Active Free Testosterone RIA." Retrieved online at: http://secure.dslabs.com/Docments//techlit/POSs/4900AA_Apr03.pdf. June 19 2004.

Appendix A

1. Wallace W.H., Kelsey T.W. "Ovarian reserve and reproductive age may be determined from measurement of ovarian volume by transvaginal sonography." *Hum Reprod.* Jun 17 2004.

INDEX

I

Inhibin, 54–59, 63–64, 66, 68, 70, 77, 84

L

L-arginine, 51
Labia, 51
LH (luteinizing hormone), 59, 84, 86
Libido, 38
Limited supply of eggs, 53, 62
Lipid levels, 46
   see also Cholesterol
Liver, 26, 32, 39, 44–45, 60–61, 72–74
   Damage, 61
Long-lasting hormone, 23

M

Melatonin, 47–48
Menopausal, 13, 15, 19, 31–32, 39, 67, 73, 83
Menopause, 13, 15–16, 18–23, 28, 30, 32–33, 35, 39, 51, 61, 67–68, 73, 83–84, 86
   Surgical, *see also* Castration
   Chemical, *see also* Castration
Menstrual cycle, 19, 30, 33, 53, 55, 60, 74, 84
Metabolism, 32, 48–49
Molecular structure, 29
Mood swings, 32
Mouth, 32
Muscle, 32, 48–49
MYC, 40–41, 43–44

N

Nails, 32
National Institutes of Health (NIH), 21, 40
Natural, 19, 21, 23, 28–29, 31, 59, 76, 78
Nervous system, 32
Nitric oxide (NO), 45, 47–48
Nitric oxide synthase (NOS), 45

O

Orgasm, 32, 50
Osteoporosis, 32, 35, 38, 46, 52, 73, 76, 82–83
   see also Bone
Ovarian dysregulation, 63
Ovarian failure, 15–16, 18, 20, 22, 30–46, 48–54, 57, 60–61, 64–65, 71–77, 79, 82, 84
Ovarian hormone deficit, 21
Ovarian Specialist, 64, 77–78, 80–81, 83
Ovarian suppression, 61
Ovaries, 15–16, 18, 20–24, 31, 33–38, 44–57, 60, 77, 83–85

P

Patch, 18–20, 26, 48, 59, 66–69, 78
Patented hormones, 28–29
Peri-menopause, 13, 30
Pharmaceutical companies, 29, 83
Pituitary, 54
Plant source, 28
Plaque, 33, 44
Pregnancy, 15
Premarin™, 15, 18, 71, 73–77

www.ingramcontent.com/pod-product-compliance
Lightning Source LLC
Chambersburg PA
CBHW071138280326
41935CB00010B/1277